Welcome to the Peace of Mind Community!

Stay Informed

Sign up for Peace of Mind's monthly newsletter for practices you can use in the classroom and information about events, training and classroom resources.

Get Support

Visit the Educators page on our website.

Prepare to Teach

You can find links to the materials you need for this curriculum on our website under "Shop."

TeachPeaceofMind.org

Questions? Comments?

We'd love to hear from you!

@PeaceofMindorg   info@TeachPeaceofMind.org

Peace of Mind Core Curriculum for Early Childhood

Peace of Mind Core Curriculum for First and Second Grade

Peace of Mind Core Curriculum for Third to Fifth Grade

Peace of Mind Curriculum for Fourth and Fifth Grade

Peace of Mind Core Curriculum for Middle School

Henry and Friends Storybook Series

Classroom Tools and Resources

TeachPeaceofMind.org

Peace of Mind Inc., Washington, D.C.
https://TeachPeaceofMind.org
Copyright 2020
ISBN 978-0-9976954-9-6
LCCN 2020914536

Cover and interior design: Schwa Design Group
Logo: Pittny Creative

Published 2020

Contents

I. Introduction

Welcome to the *Peace of Mind Core Curriculum for Middle School*. In this curriculum, we offer the practice of mindfulness not only as a means to help students calm down, but also as a skill to help them become kind and courageous peacemakers and agents of positive change.

I began teaching conflict resolution at my school in 2003. I quickly realized that my students were not able to use the skills we practiced in class when it mattered. Most of them just didn't know how to calm down enough in order to put their conflict resolution tools to work. When I began to incorporate mindfulness practices and basic neuroscience into my classes, everything changed. I was able to teach about conflict resolution and social emotional learning in a way that was deeper and more effective. This work has been transformative for my students and our school, and led us to write *The Peace of Mind Curriculum Series* to share what we know works.

Many people think that practicing mindfulness means clearing your mind. But it's actually quite the opposite: it's more about *metacognition* or "thinking about thinking."

Through mindfulness practice we notice how our mind is always flitting around finding new things to think about, almost as if there is a remote control in our brain that changes our channels randomly. We can consciously choose a channel, but then our mind might change the channel, and we might not even notice it. Sound familiar?

Mindfulness helps us to get better at noticing what is happening in our minds, and get more intentional about what we want to be thinking about. Having the ability to notice what your mind is doing and make a choice about what you want to do is liberating and powerful.

As we write this curriculum, our country is in the midst of two pandemics: COVID-19 and systemic racism. As we live in quarantine for months on end, people have also taken to the streets in huge demonstrations to protest the killing of George Floyd and many other Black people. We believe that our country and our world are at a crossroads and that mindfulness can be a powerful tool to help us find our way.

We can use mindful breathing practices to help us to deal with fear and anxiety. We can use metacognition to help us to notice when we are walking around in a fog of worry and make a different choice. These skills have helped my students and me tremendously during the COVID-19 pandemic. As you practice these skills throughout the year, they will begin to be there when you and your students need them too.

Mindfulness can also be an important tool to help us deal with structural challenges in our schools and communities, including systemic racism. Metacognition skills help us to investigate our own thoughts in order to uncover, challenge, and face our own implicit bias.

We all have implicit or unconscious bias; it is passed on from our families and through the culture. We are not responsible for having this bias. We didn't choose it. But it is our responsibility to reckon with it. And we can only do that if we know that it's there. This is work we can do ourselves and that we can help our students explore as well.

James Baldwin said, "Not everything that is faced can be changed. But nothing can be changed until it is faced." Through mindfulness practice we are able to start to see what we are thinking about other people and ourselves and then wonder: Why do I feel this way? Where does this feeling come from? Where did I hear these stories? Is this how I really feel? What can I do about it? These metacognitive skills are some of the most powerful mindfulness tools we can develop.

As much as I believe in the power of mindfulness and social emotional learning, I do have a concern. I sometimes hear mindfulness programs pitched as something that can help children "control" their emotions. Administrators are sometimes convinced to incorporate mindfulness programs like this one to help with kids who are "out of control" or in schools that have serious behavior challenges. I sometimes hear people say that mindfulness skills are especially important for "those kids." This is not what mindfulness is about.

Mindfulness is not a behavior management tool or a punishment. Children have a right to all of their emotions. Mindfulness skills can help all of our children to cope with and heal their emotions and it can also prepare them to channel their anger into righteous action to change the world, if that's what they choose.

As teachers we are all in a position to shape the minds and the hearts of our students. That is an awesome responsibility. And I believe that we owe it to our children to do our own work first. To be sure that we model and teach the skills that they will need to create the world that they deserve. A world where every child knows that they are loved and valued and safe exactly as they are. A world in which children of color are not heralded for "beating the odds" but a world in which the odds aren't stacked against them.

There is no question that we are going to make mistakes - I have made quite a few and learned from each one. We hope that learning along with your students, especially learning and using the mindfulness practices, will be a powerful way to build connections with each other.

We are all at different places in our work with social justice. Some of you might have picked up this curriculum because you are a long-time social justice educator and want to deepen the scope of your work by bringing in mindfulness. Some of you may be new to this work and will find some of these lessons challenging. Your experience teaching this curriculum will vary based on your own racialized or gender identity and your own experiences with discrimination.

There is plenty of room in the Peace of Mind Curriculum for your ideas, experiences, stories and interests, and the lessons will benefit from everything that you can bring to them. The more you are willing to share your own experiences with your students, the more they will feel safe and comfortable taking the risks that lead to growth.

Please let us know if you have questions about the *Peace of Mind Curriculum* or suggestions for us. We would love to hear from you.

We wish you happiness, health and peace.

Linda Ryden 2020

Overview

Welcome to the *Peace of Mind Curriculum for Middle School.* This curriculum teaches secular mindfulness practices, basic information about neuroscience, and an effective conflict resolution method. Over the course of the year, students will learn and practice ways to help them cope with difficult emotions and challenging situations that will be useful in school and in life.

In addition to helping students develop skills to help themselves and to become peacemakers, the *Peace of Mind Core Curriculum for Middle School* equips and inspires students to address unkindness and unfairness when they encounter it at school or with friends, and to feel confident in their capacity to contribute to making the world a better place. This curriculum includes challenging, important lessons on noticing and addressing stereotypes, recognizing and addressing implicit bias, understanding and standing up to bullying behavior, and applying all of these skills to making positive social change.

Teaching the ***Peace of Mind Curriculum*** weekly over the course of the whole school year and integrating elements of *Peace of Mind* into every day creates positive change in a classroom and, over time, in a school's climate.

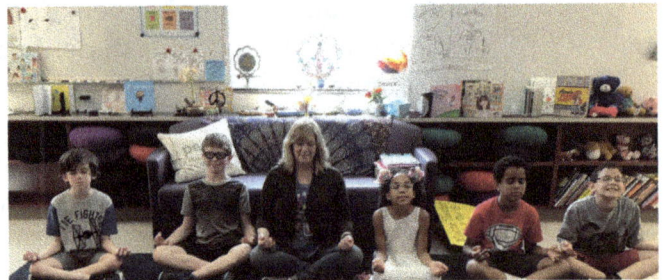

For an overview of the philosophy, history and goals of the **Peace of Mind Program**, please watch the short video introduction by Peace Teacher and curriculum author Linda Ryden on our website: TeachPeaceofMind.org/videos/.

Curriculum Structure

The ***Peace of Mind Core Curriculum for Middle School*** includes four critical, integrated components:

- **Mindfulness**
- **Brain Science**
- **Social and Emotional Learning (SEL) and Conflict Resolution**
- **Applying Mindfulness for Social Change**

Every lesson begins with mindfulness practice and ends with Peace Partner practice. Brain science, social emotional learning (SEL), conflict resolution and social justice lessons are particularly effective because they are built upon this foundation.

Mindfulness

Mindfulness is the practice of paying attention to our thoughts, our feelings, and what is happening around us, and putting some space between our reactions and our response. Mindfulness practice in this curriculum might include quietly sitting to focus on breath awareness, practicing mindful listening, noticing where our thoughts are, noticing how our bodies feel when we have different emotions, engaging in active movement, and more.

Mindfulness practice is becoming more prevalent in schools because research shows that mindfulness training can help to enhance attention and focus (Zenner et al., 2014; Zoogman et al. 2015), improve self-control and emotion regulation (Metz et al., 2013), and improve overall social emotional competence including increased empathy, perspective-taking, and emotional control, and less peer-rated aggression (Schonert-Reichl et al., 2014; Schonert-Reichl & Lawlor, 2010).

Brain Science

Teaching basic neuroscience as it relates to emotions and mindfulness is a key ingredient in **Peace of Mind**'s approach. **Peace of Mind** offers students a basic understanding of the roles of the amygdala, the hippocampus, and the prefrontal cortex in reacting and responding to stimuli. This knowledge helps students understand how and why we get angry, for example, and how and why practicing mindfulness can help us calm down enough to make a decision that moves us closer to the outcome we'd like to have. This knowledge can be liberating for our students.

Social and Emotional Learning (SEL)

SEL is the process through which we learn to manage emotions; set and achieve positive goals; feel and show empathy for others; establish and manage positive relationships; and make responsible decisions. *(CASEL.org)*

A growing body of research shows that tending to students' social and emotional needs has positive benefits. A meta-analysis of 213 school-based SEL programs with over 270,000 students found that students who received SEL instruction, compared to a control group, showed significantly improved social and emotional skills, attitudes and behavior, and an 11 percent gain in academic achievement. (Durlak et al., 2011).

Peace of Mind's SEL components include: kindness practice in every lesson through Peace Partner and lessons on empathy, gratitude practice, building connection, apologizing and solving conflicts peacefully.

Peace of Mind helps to create a kind and inclusive school culture. Creating a kinder, more positive school climate and dedicating class time for social emotional learning are two important and evidence-based approaches to bullying prevention (Bradshaw, 2015; O'Brennan & Bradshaw, 2013).

Peace of Mind's goals and lesson structure are aligned with the 5 Core Competencies identified by the Collaborative for Social and Emotional Learning (CASEL).

Peace of Mind teaches mindfulness-based Social and Emotional Learning (SEL). We know that mindfulness and SEL both have positive benefits for our students and our schools. But here's what's really exciting: we have learned in over a decade of doing this work that integrating mindfulness with SEL is an even more transformative approach than either one on its own.

Ultimately, when taught and learned together, mindfulness and SEL have the potential to transform our communities and our world with the former cultivating the tendencies for compassion and ethical ways of living and the latter teaching the skills to make that happen.

— Linda Lantieri, Senior Program Advisor for CASEL and Director of The Inner Resilience Program

Social Justice

Middle Schoolers care about the world around them and want to make a positive difference in their communities. When they are able to draw on their own mindfulness practice, an understanding of their brains, social emotional skills and the tools to solve conflicts peacefully as a foundation for social justice work, the results can be so powerful.

As educators, we have the capacity to support our students' work for a more equitable world. Dena Simmons, Director of Education at the Yale Center for Emotional Intelligence, says:

"Teaching for an antiracist future starts with us, the educators. An antiracist educator actively works to dismantle the structures, policies, institutions, and systems that create barriers and perpetuate race-based inequities for people of color. Educating students to see and respect the humanity and dignity of all people should be a national imperative, especially if we want to heal— and have a future—as a nation."

Our students and schools need what you have to give.

Lesson Themes

The 32 weekly lessons in this Curriculum are divided into 6 units and a closing lesson focused in the following areas:

Unit 1: Community Building and Introduction to Mindfulness (4 lessons)

The first four lessons focus on building community through icebreakers, community agreements and the introduction of Peace Partners. Watching and discussing the video "Under Pressure" provides context for Peace of Mind class. Foundational mindfulness practices are introduced.

Unit 2: Your Body, Your Mind, Your Feelings (5 lessons)

In this unit, we explore the embodiment of feelings and the nature of our thoughts. When we notice where feelings begin in our bodies, it gives us a head-start on gaining control over how we respond to them. When we learn to notice when our thoughts "change channel," we gain control over where we are focusing our attention.

Unit 3: Gratitude and the Negativity Bias (2 lessons)

In this unit, we explore our brain's tendency to focus on the negative and how we can balance this tendency with gratitude practice.

Unit 4: Your Brain and Your Thoughts (3 lessons)

In this unit, we review the functions and inter-relatedness of three key parts of our brains: the amygdala, the hippocampus and the prefrontal cortex. We put this knowledge to work in written reflection, role plays and skits.

Unit 5: Conflict Resolution (5 lessons)

In this unit, we introduce the concept of the Conflict Escalator, explore what makes a good apology, and meet the Conflict CAT, a method for resolving conflicts. Through discussion, skits and games, we apply what we've been learning about mindfulness, kindness, empathy, and brain science to the challenge of resolving conflicts peacefully.

Unit 6: Mindfulness for Social Justice (12 lessons)
In this unit, we explore how mindfulness practices, particularly those that help us notice our thoughts, help us to address stereotypes and implicit bias. We focus on the need for compassion for ourselves and others, and students begin to explore how they can use what they've been learning to address societal challenges.

Wrapping it Up
The final lesson of the year invites students to reflect on what they have learned and how they can put their skills to work.

> *NOTE: You might choose to follow up on the final class with a service project that allows students to put their skills to work. While this is beyond the scope of this curriculum, we hope you'll consider it! You'll find one example of such a project after the final lesson.*

Lesson Sequence

Lessons are designed to be taught in the order in which they are presented. Studies in our pilot schools suggest that teachers and students perceive the most benefit when the curriculum order is followed.

The very first lesson you teach about mindfulness is actually the first step toward peaceful conflict resolution in your classroom. From Lesson 1, you will be building the foundation that will enable students to solve conflicts with empathy, compassion and skill. Every lesson is a critical piece of the foundation for successful conflict resolution. Without the foundation, the conflict resolution lessons themselves will be less effective.

However, we know that in some cases, it may make sense to you to change the order of lessons to meet your students' needs or to coincide with events in your school community. Please do what you think best meets the needs of your class

For example, if you are seeing a great deal of conflict among your students in the beginning of the year and would like to get to those lessons more quickly, here is an alternative sequence: Teach all of Unit 1 and then go directly to Unit 4, Brain Science and then Unit 5, Conflict Resolution. After Unit 5, you can return to Units 2 and 3, and then move to Unit 6.

Most of the lessons bear repeating. If you feel your class needs more practice in a certain area, and you have the time, feel free to repeat the lesson, or segment of the lesson, that feels helpful.

Lesson Framework

Each lesson includes the following components:

- **Mindfulness and Mindfulness Leader**

  You may choose to have one Mindful Leader or a pair of Mindful Leaders lead the Mindfulness practice in each class. The role of Mindful Leader(s) will pass to new students each week. Students reinforce their own skills when they lead practices for their peers. Leadership of this part of class may be particularly beneficial for students who do not have leadership opportunities in other areas of their lives.

- **Lesson**

  Weekly lessons are designed to be engaging and challenging with a balance of listening, discussion, and activity. Some lessons focus primarily on introducing a new mindfulness practice; most start with a mindfulness practice as the foundation for topics described above.

- **Optional Role-plays and Skits**

  Role-plays and skits are included throughout the curriculum to help students practice and embody the skills and tools they are learning. Some middle schoolers really enjoy these acting opportunities and some do not. Please rely on your own judgment about whether or not to include role plays in skits for your students. We have offered other alternatives that can be done instead or in addition.

- **Peace Partners**

  Not only do Peace Partners give students a way to practice kindness, they are an essential tool for building a positive and inclusive classroom and school community. The Peace Partner practice at the end of each lesson may include:

  – Sharing what Partners did for each other in the previous week
  – Assignment of new Peace partners

- The Peace Partner Challenge: an activity that invites students to find out as much as they can about each other in 90 seconds.
- Sharing what Partners learned during the Challenge.

You may not need or have time for all of these components in every class.

> **NOTE:** *In some lessons, you'll find guidance to assign your new Peace Partners before the end of class in order to have new Partners work together on pair activities.*

Materials Needed

The only things you will definitely need for this curriculum are a means to show videos to your class and paper and writing materials for some lessons.

Optional materials include:

- a journal for each student. These may be used for written reflection in any lesson.
- a bell or a chime
- collage materials for two lessons
- *Peace of Mind* classroom resources
  - **Ways to Practice Mindfulness** - classroom poster that reminds students of the practices they've learned, and helps them to choose a practice of their own as needed.
  - **Peace of Mind Anchor Charts** for the Brain and Conflict Toolbox.
  - **The Conflict CAT Game** used in the Conflict Resolution section
  - Please visit TeachPeaceofMind.org/shop/ for a full range of classroom resources.

Teacher Guidance

The first paragraph of each lesson offers you an overview of the lesson, and some include recommended reading to prepare to teach.

All of the lessons offer suggested scripts for you. They are there if you need them. Please use them as a support, but feel free to teach the lesson in your own words in the way that feels most natural to you.

Unit 6, our unit on Mindfulness for Social Justice, invites you and your students into challenging conversations about identity, bias, race, and standing up for what you believe in. You will find resources to help you prepare to teach this section in the Social Justice Resource Section at the end of the curriculum and in the introduction to many of the lessons in Unit 6. *We recommend giving yourself plenty of time to explore these resources before you reach Lesson 20.*

Still have questions?

After reading the introductory material here, you may still feel that you would like some support preparing to teach *Peace of Mind*. You will find additional resources at TeachPeaceofMind.org/for-Educators.

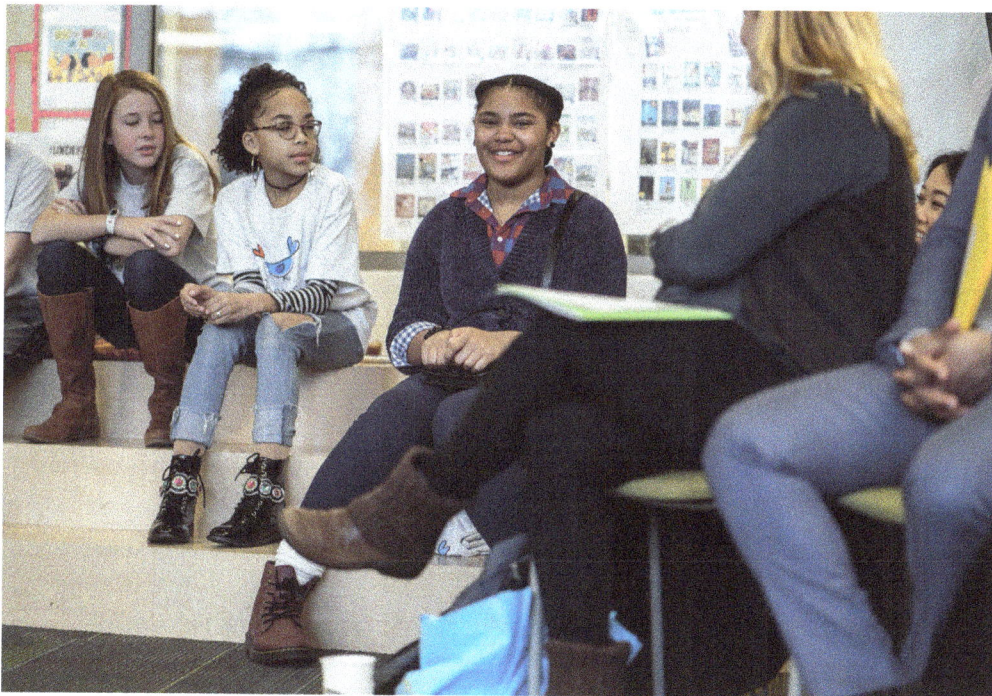

Lessons At-a-Glance

Lesson	Mindfulness Skill	Lesson Objective(s)	CASEL
1. Introduction to Peace Class	Mindful Listening	Introduce Peace of Mind Class. Engage students in mindfulness. Introduce Peace Partners to begin to form connections within the group. Establish class norms.	2, 3, 4
2. Who am I?	Balanced Breathing	Engage in self-reflection about our identities. Engage students in mindfulness. Assign new Peace Partners. Revisit class norms.	1, 2, 3, 4
3. Who are You?	Squeeze and Release	Build class community. Engage students in mindfulness. Practice kindness. Assign new Peace Partners.	1, 2, 3, 4, 5
4. THiNK Test	Four Square Breathing	Learn how to communicate mindfully. Practice thinking before you speak. Practice kindness.	1, 2, 3, 4
Unit 2 – Your Body, Your Mind, Your Feelings			
5. See, Hear, Feel	See, Hear, Feel	Learn a new way of practicing mindfulness. Practice kindness. Assign new Peace Partners.	1, 2, 3, 4
6. Visualization	Visualization	Learn the skill of visualization to calm down and focus. Practice kindness. Assign new Peace Partners.	1, 2, 3, 4
7. Find your Feelings	Recognizing Feelings	Learn to relate physical feelings to our emotions. Practice kindness. Assign new Peace Partners.	1, 2, 3, 4

Lesson	Mindfulness Skill	Lesson Objective(s)	CASEL
8. Remote Control Breathing	Remote Control Breathing	Increase awareness of when our thoughts wander. Practice noticing thoughts. Practice kindness. Assign new Peace Partners.	1,2,3,4
9. Where are your Thoughts?	Past, Present, or Future	Notice if thoughts are mostly about the past, present or future. Practice kindness. Assign new Peace Partners.	1, 2, 3, 4, 5
Unit 3 – Gratitude and Negativity Bias			
10. The Negativity Bias	Web of Gratitude	Learn about the Negativity Bias and how we can "hack" our brains to reduce its power. Practice kindness. Assign new Peace Partners.	1, 2, 3,4
11. Expressing Gratitude	Web of Gratitude	Practice Gratitude. Recognize how expressing gratitude makes you feel. Practice kindness. Assign new Peace Partners.	1, 2, 3, 4, 5
Unit 4 – Your Brain and Your Thoughts			
12. Meet Your Brain	Take 5 Breathing	Learn about three key parts of the brain. Practice kindness. Assign new Peace Partners.	1, 2, 3, 4, 5
13. Your Brain and Basketball	Student choice: Take Five, Gravity Hands, Clench and Release, Four Square, See, Hear, Feel	Introduce student choice in mindfulness practice. Deepen understanding of how parts of the brain are interrelated through the Elijah's brain skit. Practice kindness. Assign new Peace Partners.	2, 3, 4
14. Flow	Flow	Learn about the concept of flow. Explore how flow applies to students' lives. Practice a new mindfulness exercise. Practice kindness. Assign new Peace Partners.	1, 2, 3, 4, 5

Unit 5 – Conflict Resolution			
Lesson	Mindfulness Skill	Lesson Objective(s)	CASEL
15. Introduce the Conflict Escalator	Gravity Hands	Learn about what causes conflicts to escalate. Learn a new way to talk about conflict escalation. Use skits to notice when a conflict is escalating. Engage students in mindfulness. Practice kindness. Assign new Peace Partners.	1, 2, 3, 4, 5
16. MOFL or Awful (Apologizing)	Recognizing Feelings	Explore methods to de-escalate conflicts. Explore what makes a good apology. Practice apologizing. Practice kindness. Assign new Peace Partners.	1, 2, 3, 4, 5
17. The Conflict CAT	Student choice: Take Five, Gravity Hands, Clench and Release, Four Square, See, Hear, Feel	Learn and practice using the Conflict CAT to resolve conflicts. Engage students in mindfulness. Practice kindness. Assign new Peace Partners.	1, 2, 3, 4, 5
18. Conflict CAT continued	Student choice: Take Five, Gravity Hands, Clench and Release, Four Square, See, Hear, Feel	Practice using the Conflict CAT. Practice kindness. Assign new Peace Partners.	1, 2, 3, 4, 5
19. Conflict CAT Game (optional)	Student choice: Take Five, Gravity Hands, Clench and Release, Four Square, See, Hear, Feel	Practice Conflict Resolution skills. Engage students in mindfulness. Practice kindness. Assign new Peace Partners.	1, 2, 3, 4, 5
Unit 6 – Implicit Bias, Stereotypes, and Actions			
20. Compassion for Ourselves and Others	Heartfulness	Practice giving compassion to ourselves and to others. Learn the mindfulness practice Heartfulness. Practice kindness. Assign new Peace Partners.	1, 2, 3, 4, 5

Lesson	Mindfulness Skill	Lesson Objective(s)	CASEL
21. Fast and Slow Thinking	Remote Control Breathing	Learn about Fast and Slow Thinking. Engage students in mindfulness. Practice kindness. Assign new Peace Partners.	1, 2, 3, 4, 5
22. Like A What?	Remote Control Breathing	Learn about stereotypes and bias. Engage students in mindfulness. Establish terms. Practice kindness. Assign new Peace Partners.	1, 2, 3, 4, 5
23. Everybody Cries	Remote Control Breathing	Continue to explore stereotypes and bias.. Engage students in mindfulness. Establish terms. Practice kindness. Assign new Peace Partners.	1, 2, 3, 4, 5
24. Bias and Discrimination	Remote Control Breathing	Learn more about bias and discrimination. Engage students in mindfulness. Practice kindness. Assign new Peace Partners.	1, 2, 3, 4, 5
25. What is Implicit Bias?	Remote Control Breathing	Learn about implicit, or unconscious, bias. Apply knowledge of brain science to help address bias. Engage students in mindfulness. Practice kindness. Assign new Peace Partners.	1, 2, 3, 4, 5
26. Using Mindfulness to Notice Bias	Flashlight Body Scanning	Learn to use mindfulness skills to help us notice what we are thinking about others and identify implicit bias. Practice kindness.	1,2,3,4,5
27. That's Not Me	Four Square Breathing	Continue to explore bias and stereotypes. Engage students in mindfulness. Practice kindness. Assign new Peace Partners.	1, 2, 3, 4, 5

Lesson Title	Mindfulness Practice	Practice Description	
28. Counter Stereotypes	Four Square Breathing	Learn to use mindfulness skills to help us notice what we are thinking about others. Identify counter stereotypes. Practice kindness.	1, 2, 3, 4, 5
29. Speaking Up	Recognizing Feelings	Explore how to use what we've learned to stand up against unfair and unkind treatment of others. Practice kindness.	1, 2, 3, 4, 5
30. Burgers and Bullying	See, Hear, Feel	Learn how to take action when we witness or experience unkind action based on bias. Recognize the powerful role a bystander can play in bullying. Help to build the courage to stand up for yourself and others. Engage students in mindfulness. Practice kindness. Assign new Peace Partners.	1, 2, 3, 4, 5
31. Just Like Me	See, Hear, Feel	Reinforce our common humanity. Build our sense of community. Engage students in mindfulness. Practice kindness. Assign final Peace Partners.	1, 2, 3, 4, 5
Reflection and Wrapping it Up			
32. Reflection and Next Steps	Student Choice	Reflect and consider next steps. Engage students in mindfulness. Practice kindness.	1, 2, 3, 4, 5

*Correlation with the five Core SEL Competencies identified by the Collaborative for Social Emotional Learning (CASEL.org)

1. Self-Awareness
2. Self-Management
3. Social Awareness
4. Relationship Skills
5. Responsible Decision Making

Mindfulness Practices by Lesson

Unit 1 - Community Building and Introduction to Mindfulness

Lesson Title	Mindfulness Practice	Practice Description
1. Introduction to Peace Class	Mindful Listening	Listen to sounds and pay attention to them.
2. Who Am I?	Balanced Breathing	Practice mindfulness through focusing on the breath.
3. Who Are You?	Squeeze and Release	Focus on clenching one body part then releasing, moving through the whole body.
4. THiNK Test	Four Square Breathing	Draw an invisible square in the air in front of you. Imagine starting in the bottom left hand corner of a square. Breathe in and draw a line up while you slowly count to four. Hold your breath as you draw a line across the top and slowly count to four. Then breathe out as you draw a line down and slowly count to four. Then wait as you draw a line across the bottom connecting the lines of the square and slowly count to four.

Unit 2 - Your Body, Your Mind, Your Feelings

Lesson Title	Mindfulness Practice	Practice Description
5. See, Hear, Feel	See, Hear, Feel	Pay attention to three things: what we see, what we hear, and what we feel in our bodies.
6. Visualization	Visualization	Visualize a peaceful place, maybe a place you've been or a place you'd like to go. Notice how you feel there.

7. Find your Feelings - story - vocab and sensations	Recognizing Feelings	Imagine a situation such as, "you are lying in bed and you wake up and realize that it is time to go to school." Then ask "How do you feel?" and "Notice where you feel it."
8. Remote Control Breathing	Remote Control Breathing	Count your breaths. Pay attention to what happens in your mind when you try to count breaths and imagine using a remote control in the mind.
9. Where are your thoughts?	Past, Present, or Future	Notice where your thoughts take you when you try to focus on our breath. Are you thinking about the past (like something that happened last night), the future (an important game you have tomorrow), or the present (maybe how hungry you are)? Simply recognize how you feel and what you're thinking.

Unit 3 - Gratitude and Negativity Bias

Lesson Title	Mindfulness Practice	Practice Description
10. The Negativity Bias and Marble Game	Web of Gratitude	Think about people or things that you are grateful for and imagine putting them in a web of gratitude and saying "Thank you" to them.
11. Expressing Gratitude	Web of Gratitude	Think about people or things that you are grateful for and imagine putting them in a web of gratitude and saying "Thank you" to them.

Unit 4 - Your Brain and Your Thoughts

Lesson Title	Mindfulness Practice	Practice Description
12. Meet Your Brain	Take 5 Breathing	Track your breaths by tracing the outside of your fingers. Trace up one finger and breathe in, then trace down that finger and breathe out.

Lesson Title	Mindfulness Practice	Practice Description
13. Your Brain and Basketball	Student choice: Take Five, Squeeze and Release, Four Square, See, Hear, Feel	
14. Flow	Flow	Enter the "flow state" by calling on a memory of being "in the zone." Imagine the sensations in the body during this time as well as the scenery.

Unit 5 - Conflict Resolution

Lesson Title	Mindfulness Practice	Practice Description
15. Introduce the Conflict Escalator	Gravity Hands	Start with your hands on your knees with your palms facing up. As you slowly breathe in, lift your hands up just about to shoulder height and then slowly turn them over and lower them as you breathe slowly out.
16. MOFL or Awful (Apologizing)	Recognizing Feelings	Imagine a situation such as, "you are lying in bed and you wake up and realize that it is time to go to school." Ask "How do you feel?" and "Point to where you feel it."
17. The Conflict CAT	Student choice: Take Five, Squeeze and Release, Four Square, See, Hear, Feel, Gravity Hands	
18. Conflict CAT Role Play	Student choice: Take Five, Squeeze and Release, Four Square, See, Hear, Feel, Gravity Hands	
19. Conflict CAT Game (optional)	Student choice: Take Five, Squeeze and Release, Four Square, See, Hear, Feel, Gravity Hands	

Unit 6 - Implicit Bias, Stereotypes, and Actions

Lesson Title	Mindfulness Practice	Practice Description
20. Compassion for Ourselves and Others	Heartfulness	Choose someone who makes you happy, someone you may be in conflict with, and yourself and think of the words "may you be happy, healthy, peaceful."
21. Fast and Slow Thinking	Remote Control Breathing	Count your breaths. Pay attention to what happens in the mind when you try to count breaths and imagine using a remote control in the mind.
22. Like A What?	Remote Control Breathing	Count your breaths. Pay attention to what happens in the mind when you try to count breaths and imagine using a remote control in the mind.
23. Everybody Cries	Remote Control Breathing	Count your breaths. Pay attention to what happens in the mind when you try to count breaths and imagine using a remote control in the mind.
24. Bias and Discrimination	Remote Control Breathing	Count your breaths. Pay attention to what happens in the mind when you try to count breaths and imagine using a remote control in the mind.
25. What is Implicit Bias?	Remote Control Breathing	Count your breaths. Pay attention to what happens in the mind when you try to count breaths and imagine using a remote control in the mind.

26. Using Mindfulness to Notice Bias	Flashlight Body Scanning	Sitting or lying down, still so that the only thing moving is your breathing, imagine a flashlight hanging over your body that you can use to scan over different body parts. When the light is on a part of the body, focus on how that part feels, and move to the next body part.
27. That's Not Me	Four Square Breathing	Draw an invisible square in the air in front of you. Imagine starting in the bottom left hand corner of a square. Breathe in and draw a line up while you slowly count to four. Hold your breath as you draw a line across the top and slowly count to four. Then breathe out as you draw a line down and slowly count to four. Then wait as you draw a line across the bottom connecting the lines of the square and slowly count to four.
28. Counter Stereotypes	Four Square Breathing	Draw an invisible square in the air in front of you. Imagine starting in the bottom left hand corner of a square. Breathe in and draw a line up while you slowly count to four. Hold your breath as you draw a line across the top and slowly count to four. Then breathe out as you draw a line down and slowly count to four. Then wait as you draw a line across the bottom connecting the lines of the square and slowly count to four.

Lesson Title	Mindfulness Practice	Practice Description
29. Speaking Up	Recognizing Feelings	Imagine a situation such as, "you are lying in bed and you wake up and realize that it is time to go to school." Ask "How do I feel?" and "Where do I feel it?"
30. Burgers and Bullying	See, Hear, Feel	Pay attention to three things: what you see, what you hear, and what you feel in your body.
31. Just Like Me	See, Hear, Feel	Pay attention to three things: what you see, what you hear, and what you feel in your body.

Unit 7 - Wrapping it Up

Lesson Title	Mindfulness Practice	Practice Description
32. Reflection and Next Steps	Student choice: Take Five, Squeeze and Release, Four Square, See, Hear, Feel, Gravity Hands	

Engaging Middle School Students

Introducing this Curriculum

The key message we recommend sharing with your students is: These practices are tools to help you manage your own emotions, understand and control your reactions, build stronger friendships, and solve conflicts skill- fully. These tools will also support you in making the changes you want to see in the world. *This is for you.*

If you are teaching students who have had the *Peace of Mind Core Curriculum* in elementary school or are already familiar with mindfulness, recognize their experience. *The Peace of Mind Core Curriculum for Middle School* includes many of the same components as the *Peace of Mind Core Curriculum* for elementary school, but goes deeper in many areas including: the embodiment of feelings, talking about challenging social issues like racism and sexism; addressing bullying and bias. There is still so much to learn, and we are never finished practicing.

Expectations

We are not looking for perfection or final mastery from our students, but rather engagement and growth in the practice of mindfulness and kindness to others and ourselves.

Keep your expectations reasonable. Sometimes the kid who is sitting with their eyes wide open, legs jiggling, and fiddling with a pencil during mind- fulness practice is doing their very best and is benefiting greatly from the effort. The exercises in this curriculum are for the benefit of the students and a little moving around is ok as long as it is not preventing other students from practicing.

Connection

There may be students in your classroom who are reluctant to engage fully in mindfulness practice because they think it isn't cool. Some students may have a negative attitude toward mindfulness for other reasons. If this is the case, it can be very helpful to relate mindfulness to sports. Many sports teams and sports stars such as the Seattle Seahawks and Lebron James prac- tice mindfulness regularly to enhance their performance. Talking about how mindfulness practice can help us play better by helping us focus, control our temper, be more of a team player, connect our minds and bodies, and calming our nerves can be very influential to student athletes.

This can also be true of music, dance, and just about anything else that your students are interested in. Finding the relevance can be important, especially for middle school students.

You might remind your students that they always have a choice about whether to practice mindfulness or not. It is a personal practice. If they choose not to, that is fine, as long as they do not prevent their peers from practicing. Encourage them to stay with the group and just sit quietly and think about whatever they want to think about while the others are doing the mindfulness practice. Often knowing that they have the freedom to opt out will allow kids to opt in.

You might like to focus on the power these practices give us to take care of big emotions, to focus our attention, to decide how to respond to a given situation. These are skills for life, that allow your students to learn to control themselves.

When students practice these tools, they also have what they need to build stronger, more positive relationships with friends and family. They can be peace teachers in the way that they act and respond to situations and people around them. This is a powerful way to lead that is open to every student.

We can talk to our students about how the skills they will be learning will help them to pursue their social justice goals with more equanimity and skill. Mindfulness helps us understand our identity, to notice and address stereotypes and bias, and to solve conflicts with others in peaceful and effective ways.

Finally, it may help to think of yourself as planting and nurturing seeds that will mature at different times –- perhaps long after the school year is over.

Trauma Sensitive Teaching

One important area of growth in our field is in the area of trauma-sensitive mindfulness teaching. While mindfulness can be tremendously helpful for most people, for some, certain practices may trigger traumatic responses. These responses might range from discomfort and twitchiness to intense memories of a traumatic event. As teachers, our role is to notice our students' responses, to remind them that they always have a choice about whether to do a certain practice or not, to offer an alternative, to be flexible, and to seek help when we feel out of our depth.

Here are a few guidelines that we hope will be helpful:

- Remember, offering choice is essential, and can be especially helpful in engaging students.
- Offer alternatives to breathing practice. Some people find breathing practices to be triggering. If you notice a student who seems uncomfortable or who is resistant you might offer alternative practices such as See, Hear, Feel or Mindful Listening that don't involve focusing on the breath.
- Be flexible with points of focus. Invite open or closed eyes and allow some flexibility with body position and movement, as long as adaptations for one student do not compromise the ability of other students to practice.
- Reassure students they can stop a practice anytime, or choose another practice, as long as it doesn't interfere with anyone else's practice.
- Notice what is happening for your students as they practice. Check in with children who seem uncomfortable and offer a quiet alternative.
- Seek additional help if needed.

We encourage you to learn more about this area. Here are two excellent resources: *Trauma-Sensitive Mindfulness: Practices for Safe and Transformative Healing* by David Treleaven and *The Trauma Sensitive Classroom* by Patricia Jennings.

Modeling What You Teach

Students will take their cues from you. It is so important to establish your own mindfulness practice before you attempt to teach it to your students and to continue to be open to learning along with your students. You don't have to be an expert in mindfulness, but it is important to join your students on the journey.

You may have already found mindfulness resources that support you in teaching the **Peace of Mind Curriculum**. If not, please see the Resource area of the Appendix and visit the Educator section of the **Peace of Mind** website. TeachPeaceofMind.org

Talking About Challenging Topics

Some of the ground that we cover in this curriculum, particularly in Unit 6, is difficult. Talking about race, racism, gender stereotypes, and sexism are not things that most of us do often or comfortably in our society. When we avoid these topics, we do a real disservice to our children. As we write this curriculum, nationwide protests over the killing of George Floyd have swept the country. Children growing up today are especially aware of campaigns like Black Lives Matter but may be very confused about what is happening in our country and how we got here.

Many of us adults, especially white people, were raised to believe that being "color-blind' was virtuous and that it was impolite or inappropriate to talk about race. But when we say that we are color-blind, what we are really saying is that we are blind to the experiences of Black people and other people of color in our society. If we are to create a truly peaceful and equitable world we have to reckon with inequality and take a hard look at what we are doing, even inadvertently, to enable it. You might feel uncomfortable diving into these difficult issues. This is a very normal feeling. But we have to do it anyway.

NOTE FROM LINDA: *As a white woman, doing this work got easier when I did my own work first. You will find many of the resources I have learned from in our Resource Section at the end of the curriculum. We hope these resources will help you get you ready to have these incredibly important conversations with your students. Talking about racism and sexism has been difficult for me, but it has also given me a great sense of relief. It takes a lot of energy to try to ignore these challenges! We might not realize that we give up a little bit of our humanity when we ignore the suffering of others. By trying to have these hard conversations, we can begin to build a new world.*

UNIT 1
Community Building and Mindfulness

This section lays the groundwork for the year - getting to know each other, learning some basic mindfulness practices, creating community agreements, and learning how to communicate mindfully.

Lesson 1
Community Building and Mindfulness

OBJECTIVES:

Introduce Peace of Mind Class

Engage students in mindfulness

Introduce Peace Partners to begin to form connections within the group

Establish class norms

PREPARATION:

Review lesson

Prepare to show the video, being careful to choose your starting point to skip youtube ads: *"Under Pressure". Under Pressure - 2018 Version - Mindfulness in Schools - Mindfulness for Teens* https://www.youtube.com/watch?v=WJ-ZAyxHd9Y

Optional: bell or chime

Optional: student journals

Today's lesson introduces Peace of Mind Class and the foundation of every lesson: mindfulness. To help students see the relevance of this class, show the video "Under Pressure." This video features athletes and celebrities talking about how mindfulness helps them. One of the athletes is Kobe Bryant who died in a plane crash in 2019. You may want to warn your students that he will be speaking. Then we'll introduce the first mindfulness practice: mindful listening. Students begin to connect with each other through the introduction of Peace Partners. As a group, you will establish norms for Peace of Mind Class.

Introduction

Sample Script: *This year we'll be learning about a lot of things, including our brains: how they work and how they affect our behavior. We'll be learning about mindfulness: a tool we can use to help to calm our brains and learn more about our thoughts. We'll also be learning about conflicts and how to work them out skillfully and peacefully. We'll be learning about how to apply our skills to understand how we can recognize and address injustice. Most importantly, we'll be learning about ourselves and about each other.*

Every week we'll get together to practice mindfulness, explore our thoughts and emotions, and talk about real life problems and some strategies to deal with them.

This class isn't graded. It's a chance for us to hang out and learn about ourselves and each other. I hope it will be fun and relaxing and really helpful to you. This is for you. I'm looking forward to learning along with you.

Today we're going to start with an icebreaker and then we're going to establish some community agreements.

Icebreaker: This or That

Students walk to different sides of the room based on their preferences. They have to pick one.

- Would you rather have a dog or a cat?
- Would you rather be a dog or a cat?
- Would you rather eat french fries or potato chips?
- Would you rather eat carrots or celery?
- Would you rather ride a bike or a scooter?
- Would you rather be a bird or a bat?
- Would you rather live in the future or the past?
- Would you rather be able to talk to animals or speak all foreign languages?
- Would you rather explore space or the ocean?
- Would you rather be invisible or be able to fly?

Discuss

- What was that like for you?
- Were you surprised by any of your answers?
- Were any of the questions really hard for you to answer?

Community Agreements

Say: *In this class, we are going to be talking about our feelings, our thoughts, how we treat other people and how we treat ourselves. It's going to be important that everyone feels comfortable sharing their thoughts and it's important that it is okay for us to disagree respectfully.*

Ask: *Can you describe a time at school when you felt comfortable, when you felt like you mattered, when you felt respected and safe?*

Take some answers.

Ask: *What made you feel that way?*

Ask: *Can you describe a time when you felt like you could speak your truth and be brave?*

Take some answers.

Ask: *What made you feel that way?*

Take some answers.

Ask: *How can we make this a "brave space" to have hard conversations?*

Take some answers.

Ask: *What should we agree to do or not to do to make this space feel like that? Let's brainstorm some community agreements. These aren't rules but rather things that we all agree to do or not to do so that everybody feels welcome and safe to share.*

Brainstorm some agreements. Be sure to word the agreements in positive language: "We will be kind to each other" rather than "Don't be mean." Here are some possibilities if they are having a hard time:

- We'll speak one at a time and listen to each other.
- We'll be kind to ourselves and each other.
- We'll keep an open mind when we disagree.
- We'll use respectful language when we talk.

Ask: *How will we handle it if our agreements are broken?*

Brainstorm responses. Some possibilities might be:

- Say "ouch" when an agreement is broken.
- Let each other know as soon as you feel uncomfortable.
- Stop and talk about it.
- Start again.
- Reframe agreements as necessary.

Write up and post the community agreements. Refer back to them frequently and remind the students that they are fluid and can be added to as needed. Many of the lessons that follow will help to support norms like these. As the year goes on, prompt students to notice relationships between new skills and class norms.

Mindfulness Practice

You might say: *One thing we're going to be learning about this year is mindfulness. Have you heard of that before?*

Take some responses.

Sometimes people think of mindfulness as sitting on the floor and clearing your mind of all thoughts. Actually that's not it at all.

Mindfulness is a cool skill that you can learn that can help you deal with challenges a little better. Most people don't pay much attention to their minds or their brains but in this class that's going to be one of the main things we do.

Before we try a mindfulness practice of our own, let's have a look at who else uses it, and why.

Why are we talking about Mindfulness? How can it help?

Peace of Mind aims to teach students skills that will be useful to face challenges - whether they arise today at school, later at home, or in the future. This video helps students understand what mindfulness is, who uses it (athletes, celebrities, students), why and how it could help them.

Watch <u>Under Pressure</u>.

Discuss

- Why do athletes and celebrities use mindfulness / meditation?
- What pressures can you identify with?
- How do you think Mindfulness can be of help to you at school? At home?

Let's try it ourselves.

NOTE: As we mentioned in the section on Expectations on Page 23 we are not looking for perfection or final mastery from our students, but rather engagement and growth in the practices of mindfulness and kindness to others and ourselves.

Keep your expectations reasonable. Sometimes the kid who is sitting with his eyes wide open, legs jiggling, and fiddling with a pencil—but not talking—during mindfulness practice is doing his very best and is benefiting greatly from the effort. The exercises in this curriculum are for the benefit of the students and, as long as it is not preventing other students from practicing, a little moving around is ok. If it would be helpful, review suggestions for engaging your students on pages 23-26.

You might say: *Okay, so now we're going to try it. This might feel weird to you but remember that it won't be nearly as strange if we all do it together. Let's just try to keep an open mind and give it a try.*

Ask students to get into a comfortable position, sitting up a little straighter.

Invite students to close their eyes if they feel comfortable, or to find a point to focus on on the floor or in their laps. Offering this choice is very important; we want students to feel this practice is their own and that they are in control.

Invite everyone to take a deep breath.

You might say: *For the next few moments I want you to listen to the sounds around you and count inside your mind, not out loud, how many different sounds you hear.*

Try not to make any sounds yourself, just sit really still and count the sounds you hear. You might have to listen really hard to hear things. Ready? Close your eyes or look down. Okay let's start listening now…

Wait about thirty seconds or longer. You might subtly add some sounds (chair squeaking, footsteps, keys softly jingling, etc.) if the room is really quiet.

Say: *Now let's open our eyes.*

Discuss

- What did you notice?
- What did that feel like for you?
- How do you feel now?

You might say: *So that was practicing mindfulness. That was it! Just sitting there for a moment and listening to sounds and paying attention to them is called Mindful Listening. Even this short practice can calm our nervous system.*

Over the next few weeks we'll be learning practices that you'll be able to use in all sorts of situations to help you notice what you are hearing, feeling, seeing and experiencing and to calm big emotions like anger, anxiety and fear so that you can have more control over how you respond.

Let's spend the rest of the time we have today getting to know each other some more. Every week you are going to get a new Peace Partner. You'll get a chance to talk with them at the end of each class and will work with them whenever we do a partner activity. This should give us a chance to get to know each other better.

Peace Partners

Introduce Peace Partners

Say: *Every time we meet, I am going to give you a Peace Partner. Your job is to do something kind for this person between now and the next time we meet.*

Ask: *What are some examples of things you could do for your Peace partner? We're aiming for little kind things like saying "Hello" in the hall or sitting together at lunch, not buying big presents.*

Take some answers.

Say: *We have one very important rule about Peace Partners. Since one of the reasons we have Peace Partners is to help us practice being kind, I want to make sure that we start out with kindness. So when I tell you who your Peace Partner is going to be, I want you to say "okay" in a friendly way.*

When I tell you who your Peace Partner is, you might feel really happy and excited. Maybe your Peace Partner is already your really good friend, and it will be really easy to be kind to them.

But sometimes when I tell you who your Peace Partner is, you might feel differently. You might feel a little nervous or shy. And that's fine. Any way that you feel is fine. But at that moment, I want you to be kind to your Partner and say a friendly "Okay!" Your response matters.

Ask: Do you have to be friends with your Partner? **Take some answers**

No. You don't have to become friends with your Partner (although you might), and you don't even have to like your Partner. All I'm asking you to do is to find some way to be kind to them this week.

When we meet next time, you'll have a chance to share what you did for your Partner.

> **NOTE:** *Really stress the importance of the friendly "Okay." Kids are going to be embarrassed or uncomfortable and that's okay but it's really important that they don't let those feelings cause them to hurt somebody else's feelings. Stress the importance of the power of our reaction. Refer back to your Community Agreements here.*

Read through the list, saying, for example, "Sergio and Leonard are Peace Partners."

Wait for the "Okay" before moving on.

Say: *Now that you know who your Peace Partner is, you are going to find out a little more about them. Who has a question that we could ask our Peace Partner to get started?*

Listen to students' suggestions. They might suggest asking about their favorite song or favorite food or sport.

Assign Peace Partners.

Invite Peace Partners to sit next to each other and find out how many things they have in common in 120 seconds. Share out if there is time.

Closing words: *Okay our time is up for today. Thank you for a great class, everyone.*

Optional: *Let's have a nice quiet moment for the bell. If you want to, you can close your eyes, picture your new Peace Partner, and imagine yourself doing something kind for them this week.*

Lesson 2
Identity - Who am I?

OBJECTIVES:	Engage in self-reflection
	Engage students in mindfulness
	Assign new Peace Partners
	Practice kindness
	Revisit class norms
PREPARE:	Review lesson
	Paper, pencils, markers
	Sticky notes / paper for gallery walk
	Optional: bell or chime
	Optional: student journals

In this lesson, we continue to build our class community through an icebreaker and Peace Partners. We introduce a new mindfulness practice, explore the concept of identity maps and then draw one.

> *NOTE: If possible, keep copies of these maps to use again in Lesson 27.*

Building Community

You might want to start this class with either a class-wide Rock Paper Scissors Tournament, or the Knot exercise described here. Both build community, and the Knot activity targets problem-solving and critical thinking skills, along with following directions and leadership.

The Knot

- Divide the class into two teams. Tell the teams to choose two students to step apart from the group for the first part of the activity.

- Instruct the students to gently grasp the wrists of the person on either side of them until the entire group is connected.

- First, one of the two students who are not part of each group will twist the students into a human knot by verbally instructing them to walk under, step over, or rotate through other students' connected arms.

- Give the students two or three minutes to twist their respective groups.

- Then, the second of the two students who are not part of the twisted knot will try to untangle his or her group through verbal instructions. The first group to get untangled wins.

- Caution students to use care not to hurt one another. Ideally, students would not release their grip on the other students' wrists, but of course allow exceptions to avoid injury.

Mindfulness Practice

You might introduce the lesson by saying: *Do you remember last week when we did some mindful listening? We were sitting quietly and just listening to the sounds around us. We watched a video about some famous people who use mindfulness activities to help them to be happier and more successful. Today we're going to practice mindfulness in a different way.*

Today we're going to be doing a mindfulness practice called Balanced Breathing. This is a breathing practice, so we're going to be focused on our breath instead of sounds. All we are going to do is breathe in and out and try to make our inhale and our exhale be the same length.

Directions

- Sit up a little straighter in your chair.

- See if you can breathe in slowly for three beats and breathe out for three beats. Let's try it together.

- You can close your eyes if you want to or just look down into your lap to help you to concentrate. Let's try it now.

Take about 4 or 5 breaths this way.

Ask: What was that like for you?

Take a few responses.

Activity: Identity Maps

Say: *Today we'll be making Identity Maps. We'll be thinking about all of the different aspects of our identities and the roles we play. We'll use our identity maps to introduce ourselves to the group. We'll be sharing our maps later in class.*

Hand out a sheet of paper and a marker to everyone

Say: *Write your first name in big bold letters in the middle of your paper.*

*Now, let's think about what makes up our identity. Think about the **roles** you play in different parts of your life.*

In your family are you the oldest, the youngest, an uncle, aunt, sister, cousin?

At school are you a reader, writer, class clown, artist, leader?

Outside of school are you an athlete, gamer, activist, volunteer?

Now let's think about what else makes you <u>You</u>.

Think about your family structure (have a single mom, live with both parents, live with grandparents), religion, culture, heritage, musical taste, hobbies, and so on.

Directions

- Draw a line on the identity map for each role you want to include.
- At the end of each line write the word that describes that role or aspect of your identity.
- Add some adjectives to your identity map that would describe you in your different roles. Examples: Funny, cheerful, shy, kind, energetic, patient, impatient, active, loud, competitive, curious, brave...

Here are some sample identity maps[1]:

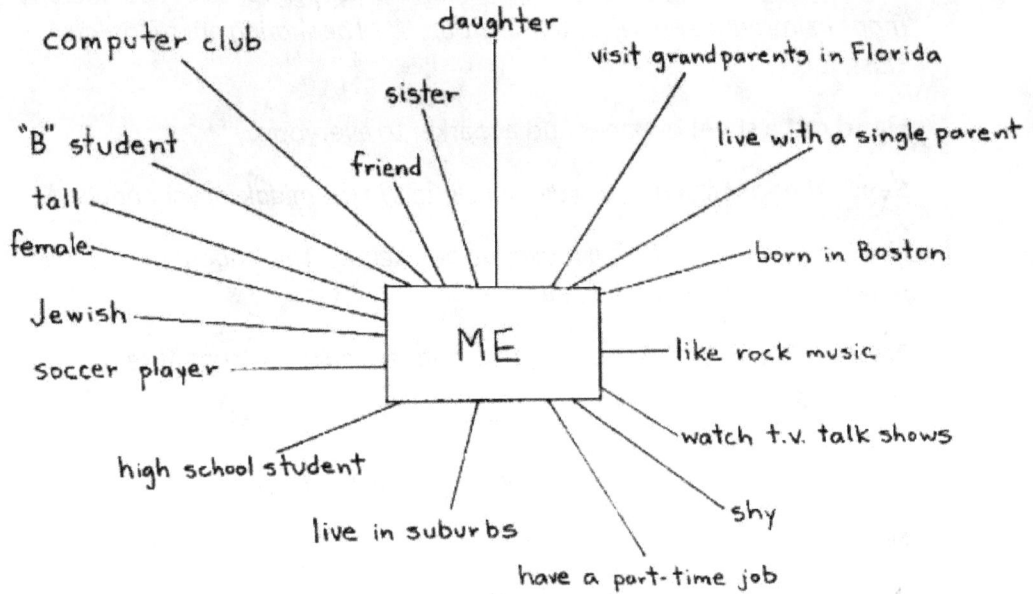

Identity map centered on a box labeled **ME** with connections to: computer club, daughter, sister, friend, visit grandparents in Florida, "B" student, live with a single parent, tall, female, born in Boston, Jewish, like rock music, soccer player, watch t.v. talk shows, high school student, shy, live in suburbs, have a part-time job.

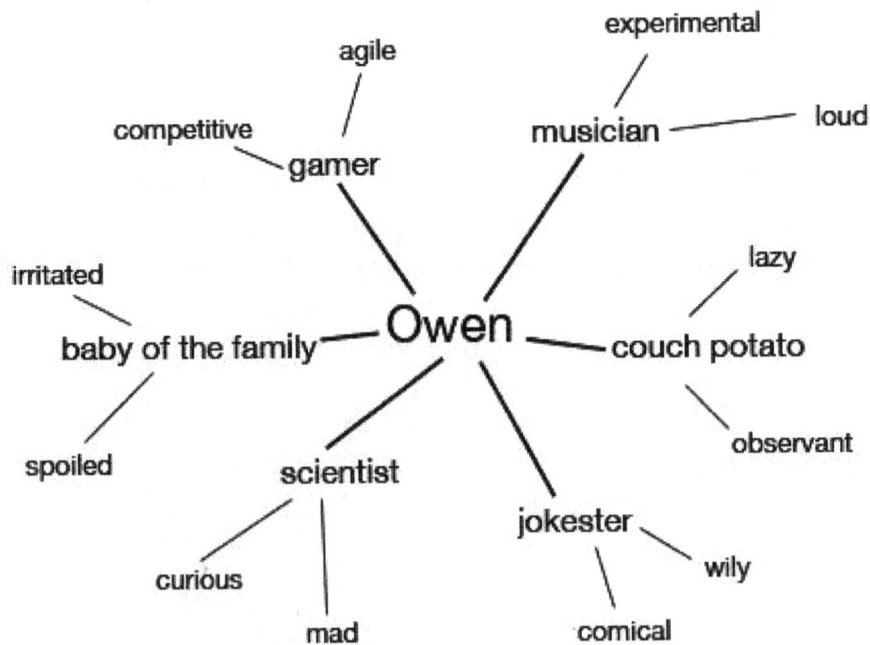

Identity map centered on **Owen** with connections to: gamer (agile, competitive), musician (experimental, loud), baby of the family (irritated, spoiled), couch potato (lazy, observant), scientist (curious, mad), jokester (comical, wily).

[1] Mapping Your Identity: A Back-to-School Ice Breaker : Lesson Plans

Sharing Identity Maps:

> NOTE: *Please make sharing identity maps optional.*

Invite students to share maps with the whole group or do a gallery walk format if they feel comfortable doing this.

Make sticky notes available.

For the gallery walk, post the identity maps on the wall and have students walk around and leave a sticky note where they find something in common.

Discuss

- Is there something that a lot of us have in common?
- Were you surprised to learn anything?
- What are some of the most important aspects of your identity to you?

Peace Partners

If there is time, give students time to share what they did for their Peace Partners over the last week.

Assign new Peace Partners. Remind your students that their job is to do at least one kind thing for their Peace Partner this week.

Closing words: *Okay our time is up for today. Thank you for a great class, everyone.*

Optional: *Let's have a nice quiet moment for the bell. If you want to, you can close your eyes, picture your new Peace Partner, and imagine yourself doing something kind for them this week.*

Lesson 3
Who are You?

OBJECTIVES:

Build class community

Engage students in mindfulness

Practice kindness

Assign new Peace Partners

PREPARATION:

Review lesson

Your Peace Partners List

Copies of *My Peace Partner's Favorite Things* worksheet

Optional: Bell or chime

Optional: student journals

Once again, we focus today on building our class community, starting with a fun group game called Count to Ten. Students will learn a new mindfulness practice and spend time interviewing their Peace Partners and creating a secret handshake.

Introduction

Say: *Last time we focused on thinking about ourselves. We mapped our identities and learned a bit about each other by sharing our maps. Today we're going to be spending more time getting to know one person—our new Peace Partner. We're going to be interviewing each other and creating a secret handshake with that person. Let's start with a fun activity.*

The Count to Ten Game

This is a fun Mindfulness game that is sometimes used in theater classes. It works here nicely because it teaches the students to listen mindfully, to focus completely on a task, to be patient with one another, and to work together as a team.

Start out with the kids sitting close together if possible. Tell everyone that they are going to try to count to ten as a group.

Say: *Today we are going to try to count to ten as a group. That sounds easy but it's actually pretty hard. Here's how it goes:*

Directions

- Close your eyes and listen carefully.

- At some point, one of you will say "one" and then someone else will say "two," and we'll keep going until we get to ten.

- Every time I hear two of you say a number at the same time, you'll have to start all over again.

- To make the game work, you are going to have to listen very carefully to each other.

- You are also going to have to be mindful of not taking too many turns.

- You also have to be mindful of making sure that you participate.

- If we get to ten, we can keep going.

- To start things out, I will say, "Start and go." Every time I hear two of you say a number at the same time I will say, "Start again and go."

- Please don't make a lot of noise when that happens. Just take a deep breath and start over again. Ready to try it?

Say: *Ok, as soon as I say go, the game starts. Someone will say "one," and we'll go from there.*

> *NOTE: This game is harder than it sounds. Encourage the students to be patient and kind with each other. There will of course be kids who want to say all the numbers who might need gentle reminders not to dominate the game, and there will also be those who will need encouragement.*

Mindfulness Practice

Say: *Today we're going to learn another way of doing mindfulness that can help you when you get angry or tense. It's called Squeeze and Release. All you do is squeeze or tighten up a part of your body—like your hands—as you breathe in and then release or relax them as you breathe out. Let's try it.*

Invite your students to:

- Sit up a little straighter.

- Close their eyes or look down.

- Take three deep breaths.
- Squeeze up one part of your body -- perhaps shoulders or hands -- and then release.
- Squeeze up another part of your body -- perhaps legs or feet -- and then release.
- Squeeze up one more part of your body - perhaps your forehead or your stomach, and then release.
- Take three deep breaths.
- Slowly open your eyes or look up.

Ask: What was that like for you?

Take a few answers.

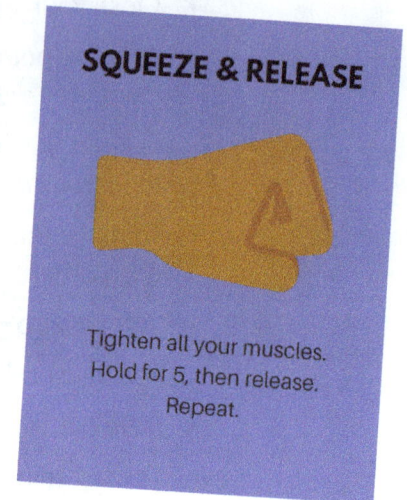

SQUEEZE & RELEASE

Tighten all your muscles.
Hold for 5, then release.
Repeat.

Peace Partners

Say: *So last time we got to know each other and ourselves. Today you're going to interview your new Peace Partner. Before I assign your new partner, would anybody like to share what they did for their Peace Partner last week? Remember you were supposed to do something kind for that person.*

Take some answers.

Assign New Partners. Remind the students to say "Okay" in a friendly way.

Hand out the " My Peace Partner's Favorite Things" worksheet.

Have the students sit with their Peace Partner. Go over the questions on the worksheet and make sure everyone understands the questions.

Directions:

- When I say go, you are going to start to interview each other. You can take turns asking each other questions (What is your Favorite movie?) and then go on to the next question.
- Sometimes people get stuck on thinking of a favorite thing. If you don't have a favorite book or movie or food just name one that you really like.
- Try to share the "Whys." Why do you like spaghetti? Try to listen really carefully to your partner's answers. We aren't going to write the answers down. Try to remember some of what your partner tells you.

- When we are finished with the interviews, I'm going to ask you to share some of what you learned about your Partner.

This might take 15-20 minutes although some kids will be done quickly. If kids are done too quickly, you might ask them to think of some bonus questions, offer some additional questions yourself, or ask them to go more into the "whys."

Share: Go through each question on the sheet and ask for some students to share what they learned about their Partner.

Ask: *Was anybody surprised about what they learned about their Partner? Did you find out that you had things in common that were unexpected?*

Secret Handshakes

This is a fun activity to help Peace Partners get to know each other and to reinforce the idea that it is possible to be kind to and have fun with students who may not be your friends. Feel free to use this activity as an icebreaker for future lessons or anytime you think it would be helpful to build relationships within your class.

Say: *Now you and your Peace Partner are going to create a secret handshake. Your handshake will demonstrate what you two have in common.*

Directions:

- You'll have ten minutes (or less if they're done sooner) to come up with your handshake and then we're going to share them with the group.
- Your handshake has to include two things: (1) words, including at least <u>five</u> things that you have in common, and (2) at least <u>five</u> movements.
- If there is an uneven number or someone is absent there can be groups of 3.

Share the handshakes with the class.

Closing words: *Okay our time is up for today. Thank you for a great class, everyone.*

Optional: *Let's have a nice quiet moment for the bell. If you want to, you can close your eyes, picture your new Peace Partner, and imagine yourself doing something kind for them this week.*

Lesson 3

Your Peace Partner's Favorite Things

Your Name: _____

Your Peace Partner's Name: _____

My Partner's favorite movie: _____

My Partner's favorite book: _____

My Partner's favorite place to visit: _____

What my Partner likes MOST about school: _____

What my Partner likes LEAST about school: _____

My Partner's favorite food: _____

My Partner's favorite singer/musician: _____

My Partner doesn't like it when people: _____

My Partner loves it when people: _____

When my Partner grows up they would like to be: _____

My Partner wishes the world were more: _____

My Partner is worried about: _____

The person/s my Partner admires the most is: _____

If my Partner could meet anyone it would be: _____

My Partner always laughs when: _____

One word to describe my Partner is: _____

Lesson 4
Mindful Communication: The THiNK Test

OBJECTIVE: Learn how to communicate mindfully

Practice thinking before you speak

Practice kindness

PREPARE: Your Peace Partners list

Board/flip chart with this quote written clearly for all to read:

> "Before you speak, ask yourself if what you are about to say is true, is helpful, is necessary, is kind. If the answer is no, then maybe what you are about to say should be left unsaid."

Optional: Prepare to watch video of Marleigh, a student, teaching Four Square Breathing. https://youtu.be/AomOaE1M9qU

Optional: bell or chime

Optional: Tyaja Uses the Think Test by Linda Ryden https://youtu.be/Rwytp7ZxDNY

Today we are introducing a new role found in all future lessons: the Mindful Leader. Each week you will choose one or two students to help lead the mindfulness practice at the beginning of class—the Mindful Leader(s). You may support the Mindful Leader(s) however they need supporting in leading the class.

We'll then learn a practice that will help students build positive relationships: the THiNK test. Over the course of the year, students will be invited to share some personal and sometimes difficult thoughts and reactions. It's important to think about how we use our words. We hope that Peace Partners and the THiNK test will be effective tools all year long to help you develop a kind and inclusive school climate.

Introduction

Introduce the role of Mindful Leader.

You might say: *Today we are going to start a new practice of having one or two of you help to lead the Mindfulness Practice. The Mindful Leader(s) will lead us in the beginning of the practice by saying, "Let's sit up a little straighter; Let's close our eyes or look down; let's take three deep breaths."*

You might say: *Today we're going to be learning a new mindfulness practice called Four Square Breathing. Deep breathing can help us to slow down or calm down and think more clearly. We'll be learning more about how that works a little later this year. We'll be learning a bunch of different mindfulness practices in this class so that you can decide what works best for you. We're all different and what helps us to focus and calm down is different for each of us.*

So let's try out Four Square Breathing.

NOTE: You may lead the practice yourself, or you could show this video of Linda's student Marleigh leading the practice. Once your students become familiar with the practices, they will be able to lead them in their own words. It is wonderful to see their skills progress!

Mindfulness Practice

Show the video of Marleigh leading Four Square Breathing if you choose: https://youtu.be/AomOaE1M9qU

Say: *Four Square breathing is another way to take deep breaths to help you to calm down. To do Four Square breathing, draw an invisible square in the air in front of you. Imagine that you are starting in the bottom left hand corner of your square. As you breathe in you draw a line up while you slowly count to four. Then you hold your breath as you draw a line across the top and slowly count to four. Then you breathe out as you draw a line down and slowly count to four. Then you wait as you draw a line across the bottom connecting the lines of the square and slowly count to four.*

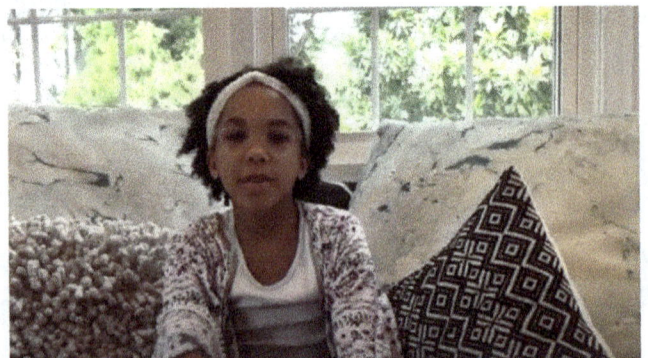

Invite the Mindfulness Leader(s) (ML) to come to the front of the class.

Prompt the ML to say: "Let's sit up a little straighter. Close your eyes or look down into your lap. Let's take 3 deep breaths."

Then you might say: *Okay let's try doing Four Square Breathing. We'll do it together. Remember you're just drawing or imaging a square as you breathe in for 4 beats, hold your breath for 4 beats, breathe out for four beats, and wait for four beats.*

Let's try it: *Breathe in 1,2,3,4 (count slowly)*

Hold your Breath 1,2,3,4

Breathe out 1,2,3,4

Wait 1,2,3,4

Repeat 2 or 3 times.

Say: *Let's take one big deep breath and reach your arms up over your head as you breathe in and slowly float them down as you breathe out.*

Say: *Now let's take one more deep breath in and then open your eyes if you have closed them.*

Optional: Ask the ML to ring the bell.

Ask the ML to return to their seat(s).

Discuss

- What was that like for you?
- Was it harder to hold your breath when your lungs were full or to wait to breathe in when your lungs were empty?

Lesson: The THiNK Test

Say: *Today we are going to be thinking about how we talk to each other. Have you ever said something and then right away wished that you hadn't said it? That has probably happened to all of us. Today we're going to learn a little trick that can help us to think before we speak so we don't end up saying things that we later regret.*

Point out this quote you have written on the board:

"Before you speak, ask yourself if what you are going to say is true, is kind, is necessary, is helpful. If the answer is no, maybe what you are about to say should be left unsaid."

Read more at: https://www.brainyquote.com/quotes/bernard_meltzer_157511

Have a few students read the quote from the board, one at a time. See if they can do it from memory.

Ask the students what the quote means to them. Take a few answers.

Introduce the THiNK test.

Suggest to the students: *This is a great quote, but it's easier when it's broken down into the THiNK Test. This stands for:*

T: true

H: helpful

N: necessary

K: kind.

Write THiNK on the board across in big letters and then write the words TRUE, HELPFUL, NECESSARY, KIND going down from the top under the corresponding letter.

Add the "I", which stands for "I" as in "I THiNK before I speak."

Talk about ways and times to use the THiNK Test.

Say: *Suppose you want to tell everyone you are eating lunch with that you are going to a party this weekend. First ask yourself, does it pass the THINK test?*

Talk about how the answer might be different if everyone you are eating lunch with is invited or only a few kids are invited.

Discuss these scenarios too:

- You want to tell someone in your class that you don't like their new haircut.
- You want to tell someone that her shoes are out of style.
- You just saw your friend bullying a younger kid.

Role Plays or Reflection

The THiNK test invites kids into thinking about ethical dilemmas. Practice really helps to understand how to apply this tool. Remember that there may not be a right or wrong answer; the point is to grapple with the choice and to think before you speak.

This activity asks students to evaluate a list of statements below using the THiNK test. Please feel free to add and use your own scenarios that may be more relevant to your students.

You have a few options here: role-playing, discussion, or written reflection - or any combination.

Discussion or written reflection

If you decide to have a discussion or to have the students respond in writing, read the following statements to your students. Ask them to evaluate each statement using the THiNK Test. Students might work individually, in pairs, or in small groups. Invite them to share their thoughts.

Remind your students that there may not be a right or wrong answer. The important thing is to consider the impact of what you are about to say before you say it.

Role-plays

If you opt for the role-plays:

- Choose four kids to represent the different words: Mr. True, Ms. Helpful, Mr. Necessary and Ms. Kind.
- Ask the group of four to try to answer these and similar questions.
- Each character will have a chance to respond to the dilemma based on their role. (Mr. True will evaluate if the statement is true, Ms. Helpful will evaluate whether the statement is helpful, and so on.).
- The class can then try to decide what course of action to take. Sometimes the answer will depend on time, place, tone of voice or other factors.
- **Repeat** with a new group of four students for each question.

Statements to evaluate with the THiNK Test

- I want to tell someone in my choir that their voice is bad.
- I want to tell everyone that I got 100% on the test.
- I want to tell someone that I just heard that "Ellen" likes "Fred."
- I want to tell someone that the TV show they like is for babies.
- I want to tell someone that their favorite YouTuber is inappropriate.
- I want to tell my parents that my friend is getting bullied, but my friend told me not to tell anyone.
- I want to tell someone that his zipper is unzipped.
- Someone is spreading a rumor that I like "Ernie" and I want to set the record straight that I don't like him.

    Ask for more examples or take their questions.

Peace Partners

Give students time to share what they did for their Peace Partners over the last week.

Assign new Peace Partners. Remind your students that their job is to do at least one kind thing for their Peace Partner this week.

Closing words: *Okay our time is up for today. Thank you for a great class, everyone.*

Optional*: Let's have a nice quiet moment for the bell. If you want to, you can close your eyes, picture your new Peace Partner, and imagine yourself doing something kind for them this week.*

UNIT 2
Your Body, Mind and Feelings

In this unit, we explore the embodiment of feelings and the nature of our thoughts. Noticing where feelings begin in our bodies gives us a head-start on controlling how we respond to them. When we learn to notice when our thoughts "change channel," we can gain control over where we are focusing our attention.

Lesson 5
See Hear Feel

OBJECTIVES: Learn a new way of practicing mindfulness

Practice kindness

Assign new Peace Partners

PREPARATION: Review lesson

Your Peace Partners list

Optional: bell or chime

Optional: student journals

Today we introduce a new Mindfulness practice called "See Hear Feel." This practice engages all of the students' senses by asking them to notice first what they see (with eyes open or closed); then what they hear in the environment; and then what they feel in their body (physical sensations). We're also going to play a mindful moving game called Walk, Stop, Wiggle, Sit.

These activities may need to be modified if there are students in your class with hearing challenges or who are differently abled. In See Hear Feel the "seeing" and the "feeling" are both internal. We are focused on what we are "seeing" in our minds and what sensations we are feeling in our bodies. However, some students may not be able to hear sounds around them. You might choose to substitute something else (smelling, for example) or just skip the hearing step for that student.

Introduction

Say: *Today we are going to try a new mindfulness practice called See Hear Feel. See, Hear, Feel is another way of doing mindfulness. Unlike the practices we've been doing so far, it isn't so much about helping us to calm down. See Hear Feel is more about helping us to pay attention.*

In this practice we are just going to be paying attention to three things: what we see, what we hear, and what we feel in our bodies. We'll be sitting quietly with our eyes closed or looking down at the floor or our laps. When I say "See" you're just going to try to notice what you are seeing.

Let's try that now: Just close your eyes or look down at the floor or your lap. What are you seeing right now? If your eyes are closed you might see lights or shapes or you might see images of things you were looking at or thinking about. (wait about five seconds) *What did you see?*

Take some answers.

Next I will say "Hear" and you can notice all of the sounds that you hear.

Let's try that now: close your eyes again or look down and try to keep your body really still so that you aren't making any noises. (Wait about five seconds) *What did you hear?*

Take some answers.

Say: *Next I will say "Feel." Try to notice feelings or sensations in your body. Sensations are physical feelings you have in or on your body. You might have an itch that you want to scratch or your hand might feel tingly. Your stomach might feel hungry or you might feel like you need to go to the bathroom.*

Those are all sensations in your body. Sensations are different but often related to emotions. Right now we are trying to focus on the sensations or body feelings.

Let's try that now: Let's close our eyes again or look down and try to keep your body really still. (Wait about five seconds) *What did you feel?*

Take some answers

So that's how you do See, Hear, Feel. So let's put it all together.

Mindfulness Practice

Invite today's Mindful Leader(s) (ML) to come to the front of the class.

Prompt the ML to say: "Sit up a little straighter. Close your eyes or look down into your lap. Let's take 3 deep breaths."

Teacher Says: *Let your breath settle back into its natural rhythm. You don't have to change it at all.*

Say: *So remember, all I am going to say is See, Hear or Feel. You're going to try to move your attention around to focus on those things that you see, hear and feel.*

Don't worry if you get distracted and start thinking about something else. That's totally normal. As soon as you notice that your mind went somewhere else just try to start again. This might happen a bunch of times and that's fine.

See… wait about ten seconds

Hear…. wait about ten seconds

Feel…. wait about ten seconds

Repeat this two or three times - if the students seem restless cut it shorter.

Okay, great job! Let's take one big deep breath and reach your arms up over your head as you breathe in and slowly float them down as you breathe out.

Optional: Ask the ML to ring the bell.

Ask the students to open their eyes and/or look up.

Ask the ML return to their seat(s).

Discuss

- Students share with their neighbor what they each saw, heard and felt.
- Direct them to take turns: first one person shares what they saw, and then the other. Then repeat with Hear and Feel.

Stop, Walk, Wiggle, Sit

Say: *Here is a new brain game that challenges our brains and challenges us to be more flexible and responsive. It also gets us moving.*

Directions

- There are many levels of this game. In each level, see if you can follow my directions.
- We're going to play the game silently so that everyone can hear the directions.
- Make sure that you are not talking and that you are not touching each other.

Level 1: When I say walk, you walk. When I say stop, you Stop. When I say wiggle, you wiggle. When I say sit, you sit. Got it?

Level 2:   Walk = Stop
           Stop = Walk
           Wiggle = Wiggle
            Sit = Sit

Level 3:   Walk = Stop
           Stop = Walk
            Wiggle = Sit
           Sit = Wiggle

Level 4:   Walk = Wiggle
           Wiggle = Walk
           Sit = Stop
           Stop = Sit

You can keep going, changing up the commands or add in new ones. It's pretty hard!

Reflect

- What was the hardest thing about this game?
- Why do you think it is hard for our brains to "go" when someone says "stop?"
- Do you think this game is challenging to your brain?
- Did your brain get used to doing different things after a while?

Peace Partners

Give students time to share what they did for their Peace Partners over the last week.

Assign new Peace Partners. Remind your students that their job is to do at least one kind thing for their Peace Partner this week.

Closing words: *Okay our time is up for today. Thank you for a great class, everyone.*

Optional: *Let's have a nice quiet moment for the bell. If you want to, you can close your eyes, picture your new Peace Partner, and imagine yourself doing something kind for them this week.*

Lesson 6
Visualization

OBJECTIVE: Learn a practice to help calm down and focus

Practice kindness

Assign new Peace Partners

PREPARE: Review the lesson

Your Peace Partners list

Prepare to show this Peace of Mind Visualization video, being careful to choose your starting point to skip YouTube ads: https://youtu.be/sW_3-ugpH80

Optional: bell or chime

Optional: student journals

Visualization is a fun way to practice mindfulness that students really enjoy. Focusing your mind on a peaceful place can help you to calm down, to focus your mind, to think about your senses, and to really settle yourself into the moment, even if it is in your imagination.

Please consider the composition of your class when you offer examples of Peaceful Places a student might call to mind. A Peaceful Place could be a real place, an imaginary place, a vacation memory, or a local park.

For this practice you can lead the visualization from the following script or you can play the video referenced above.

Introduction

You might say: *Today we're going to do a new mindfulness practice called Visualization. We're going to be focusing on a peaceful place - maybe someplace you've really been or someplace you'd like to go. It can be real or imaginary. Inside or outside. It's up to you.   This is a way to help us feel calm and peaceful.*

Mindfulness Practice

Invite today's Mindful Leader(s) (ML) to come to the front of the class.

Prompt the ML to say: "Let's sit up a little straighter. Close your eyes or look down into your lap. Let's take 3 deep breaths."

Say: *Let your breath settle back into its natural rhythm. You don't have to change it at all.*

Guide your students through a visualization exercise.

Either play the Peace of Mind Visualization Video above for the class or use this script.

Today we are going to be thinking about a Peaceful Place. Try to think about a place where you have felt really peaceful. It can be a real place, a place you've been to on vacation, your own backyard, or a place in your imagination.

Give them a moment to think.

Now let's travel to this peaceful place. Take a look around at your Peaceful Place. Are you inside or outside? What is the weather like? What can you see there? Are there trees? Is there water? If you are in a room, what color are the walls? Look around and really try to notice everything that you can see in your Peaceful Place.

Take another look around and see what you might have missed.

Pause.

Now I'd like you to listen closely. What sounds do you hear in your Peaceful Place? Do you hear birds, or the sound of the waves crashing into the shore? Do you hear people talking? Music? What else do you hear?

Pause.

What does it smell like in your Peaceful Place? Do you smell salty air? Sunscreen? Freshly cut grass? Cookies baking? What else do you smell in your Peaceful Place?

Pause.

What can you feel with your body in your Peaceful Place? Do you feel sand under your feet and between your toes? Do you feel water? Is it cold or warm? Can you feel the sun on your face? Do you feel a soft blanket? What else do you feel in your Peaceful Place?

Pause.

What does it feel like in your heart to be in your Peaceful Place? What kind of peaceful feeling do you have? Happy, safe, welcome, relaxed? Try to notice how you feel in your heart in your Peaceful Place.

Pause.

Now we are going to travel back to this peaceful place right here in our classroom.

Optional: Ask the ML to ring the bell.

Say: Open your eyes or look up when you are ready.

Ask the ML to return to their seat(s).

Discuss

- Does anybody want to share a little bit about what your Peaceful Place was like?
- What was this experience like for you?
- How do you think it could help you calm down or focus?

Peace Partners

Give students time to share what they did for their Peace Partners over the last week.

Assign new Peace Partners. Remind your students that their job is to do at least one kind thing for their Peace Partner this week.

Closing words: *Okay our time is up for today. Thank you for a great class, everyone.*

Optional: *Let's have a nice quiet moment for the bell. If you want to, you can close your eyes, picture your new Peace Partner, and imagine yourself doing something kind for them this week.*

Lesson 7
Find Your Feelings

OBJECTIVES: Learn to relate physical feelings to our emotions

Practice kindness

Assign new Peace Partners

PREPARATION: Review lesson

Your Peace Partners list

Optional: bell or chime

Optional: student journals

Today we are going to help kids locate the physical sensations of emotions in their bodies through a story. In case you would like to offer your students extra practice, we've included two optional activities as well. When kids are discussing emotions in this lesson, it might be helpful to point out:

- *Excitement* is a clenched, upward emotion. We tend to gasp when we are excited.

- *Anger* is a clenched and downward emotion. Our bellies feel tight and uncomfortable; we sometimes make fists.

- *Excitement and anger* feel similar in some ways. You might ask students to point out how they feel similar and how they feel different.

- *Sadness* is a downward emotion. Our bodies are not clenched but it's not a relaxed feeling either. Point out expressions like "feeling down" or "down in the dumps." Sadness feels low energy whereas excited feels high energy.

- *Happy* is usually a relaxed, open, pleasant feeling. There's no tightness in the belly and we're likely to have relaxed breathing.

- Sometimes kids confuse happiness with being overjoyed or excited. Ask children to point out the differences in how these emotions feel in their bodies.

- *Nervous* is a down and clenched feeling. Point out expressions like "butterflies in your stomach."

Understanding the language of our bodies can be a powerful tool to help us navigate our responses to challenging situations and emotions.

Introduction

Say: *Today we are going to explore where we feel emotions in our bodies. For example, when I feel angry, I feel it here.*

Point to where you are most aware of your own anger. **Show** where you feel excitement, sadness, nervousness, happiness in your own body.

You might say: *Not everyone will feel the same emotion in their bodies in exactly the same way. It's our job to learn our own body's language so that we can take care of our own needs and understand ourselves.*

Ask: *Where do you feel happiness?*

Take a few answers, and highlight answers that are not the same.

Ask: *Where do you feel anger?*

Take a few answers, and highlight answers that are not the same.

Ask: *Why is it important to notice where we feel emotions in our bodies?*

Take a few answers, and then explain:

One of the reasons to notice where we feel emotions in our bodies is that it can help us to take care of our emotions.

When we don't notice a feeling like anger or sadness, it can get bigger and bigger and possibly cause us to take actions that don't make things better.

Our bodies often give us the first clue to what emotion we are feeling. If we learn to pay attention to what we are noticing in our bodies, we can often understand more quickly what emotion we are having.

If you can notice, for example, anger when it is just a small feeling in your belly or a small clench of the fists, then you can use your mindful breathing skills to take care of it.

*Here's an important thing to understand: **we're not trying to get rid of our emotions; we're just trying to take care of them**. If we can notice that we're angry or sad or nervous when those feelings are small, then we can take steps to do something about what is making us feel that way. Our bodies can help us notice.*

Today we're going to do our mindfulness practice in a different way. I'm going to tell you a story and I'd like you to imagine that you are the main character in the story and try to notice your feelings.

Mindfulness Practice

Invite today's Mindful Leader(s) (ML) to come to the front of the class.

Prompt the ML to say: "Let's sit up a little straighter. Close your eyes or look down into your lap. Let's take 3 deep breaths."

The Story

Say: *Today I am going to tell you a story. I want you to imagine that you are the main character in the story and imagine how you would feel.*

Try to notice where you feel emotions in your body. For instance, if you feel mad in the story, you might point to your eyebrows or your mouth or your belly.

Don't worry if you don't notice anything. Just give it a try. There are no right or wrong answers. Remember, I am going to be asking you questions but you are going to answer them silently in your mind. We will share our answers when we are finished with the story.

Say:

Imagine that you are lying in bed and you wake up and realize that it is time to go to school. How do you feel? Where do you feel it?

You're about to get up when you remember that it's Saturday. How do you feel? Where do you feel it?

You decide to go back to sleep and you snuggle up and get comfy. How do you feel? Where do you feel it?

Suddenly you remember that you are going to meet your friends in the park today; it's your best friend's birthday. How do you feel? Where do you feel it?

You look out the window and notice that it is raining. How do you feel? Where do you feel it?

You decide to get up and read for a little while. You're in the middle of a really good book. How do you feel? Where do you feel it?

But you can't find your book anywhere. How do you feel? Where do you feel it?

You remember that your sister said that she really wanted to read that book. How do you feel? Where do you feel it?

You decide to go find your sister and demand your book back. How do you feel? Where do you feel it?

When you get out of bed you trip over your book. How do you feel? Where do you feel it?

You get up and walk into the kitchen. Your family is eating breakfast. There are pancakes for breakfast. How do you feel? Where do you feel it?

You accidentally drop a pancake and your dog drags it away to eat in her dog bed. How do you feel? Where do you feel it?

Your mom says that she has to work and can't drive you to the park. How do you feel? Where do you feel it?

You go to your room to get dressed but you can't find your lucky sweatshirt that you like to wear almost every day. How do you feel? Where do you feel it?

Your brother says that you can wear his team jersey if you want. How do you feel? Where do you feel it?

You walk to the park and the sun suddenly comes out. How do you feel? Where do you feel it?

Your friend really likes the present you made for him. How do you feel? Where do you feel it?

That's the end of the story. Let's ring the bell and then you can open your eyes and sit up and we'll share how we felt during the story.

Optional: Ask the ML to ring the bell.

Ask the students to open their eyes or look up when they are ready.

Ask the ML return to their seat(s).

Discuss

- **Go through the story again** and give one or two kids a chance to share how they felt and where they felt it at each point in the story.
- **Ask** for different reactions. It's interesting to see how kids can have completely different emotional responses to the same events. Be sure to remind them that any way that they feel is fine.

Connecting our emotions to sensations in our bodies

Following are two different activities to help students learn about the link between emotions and sensations in the body. You can decide to do one or both. What do your students need? It's up to you.

Activity 1: Act our Feelings

Explain that you are going to invite volunteers to come to the front of the class and you will whisper an emotion to them.

Emotions to act out: angry, sad, happy, scared, excited, nervous, grouchy, cheerful, relaxed, confident, confused, embarrassed, shy, silly, proud, discouraged, jubilant, enraged, panicky, miserable, terrified, ecstatic.

Invite students to act out the emotion you whisper to them by saying "Today is Tuesday" (or whatever day it is) using their body and their voice to convey the emotion. The other students will try to guess what emotion they are portraying.

> *NOTE: Some of these emotions are complex and might be new words for your students. Take some time to define the words and list them on the board if that would be helpful.*

Help kids focus on what they see in each other's bodies that give them a clue.

Ask them to point out the similarities and differences between emotions such as excited, nervous and scared.

Activity 2: Emotion vs. Sensation

Say: *In this activity, we're going to be focusing on how some of these emotions feel in our bodies.*

Draw the following on the board. Have the kids brainstorm two lists - one of emotions and one of sensations.

<u>**Emotions**</u>   <u>**Sensations (in your body)**</u>

Invite the students to see if they can make connections between the emotions and the related sensations.

You might say: *What sensations do you feel in your body when you are angry? You might feel an emotion in more than one part of your body. So one emotion might have more than one sensation. Two emotions might share the same sensation.*

Draw a line connecting the emotion on the left with all of the sensations that students suggest they feel.

Example:

Emotions	_Sensations_
Angry	upturned corners of mouth
Nervous	clenched fists
Scared	stomach ache
Excited	butterflies in the stomach
Happy	warm and tingly
Impatient	tight throat
Calm	

Peace Partners

Give students time to share what they did for the Peace Partners.

Do the Peace Partner activity as before.

Assign new Peace Partners. Remind your students that their job is to do at least one kind thing for their Peace Partner this week.

Closing words: *Okay, our time is up for today. Thank you for a great class, everyone.*

Optional: *Let's have a nice quiet moment for the bell. If you want to, you can close your eyes, picture your new Peace Partner, and imagine yourself doing something kind for them this week.*

Lesson 8
Remote Control Breathing

OBJECTIVES: Increase awareness of when our thoughts wander

Learn about metacognition

Practice noticing thoughts

Practice kindness

Assign new Peace Partners

PREPARATION: Review lesson

Your Peace Partners list

Copies of the "Remote Control" worksheet found at the end of this lesson for each student

If you choose, prepare to show Peace of Mind's Remote Control Breathing video, taking care to avoid YouTube ads: https://youtu.be/b8tQt4wovDU

Optional: bell or chime

Optional: student journals

This lesson helps students notice their thoughts and make choices about which thoughts they want to focus on and which ones they want to let go of. This awareness of what our mind is doing is called metacognition. Throughout this curriculum we will be helping students to learn how to pay attention to what their minds are doing, developing the skill of metacognition.

This lesson introduces a mindfulness practice called Remote Control Breathing, a practice that helps with metacognition. We will return to this mindfulness practice many times in the rest of the curriculum.

You might like to watch Peace of Mind's Remote Control Breathing video before you teach this practice. Feel free to share this with your class if you think it would be helpful. https://youtu.be/b8tQt4wovDU

When we recognize our thoughts, we have the opportunity to control our thoughts rather than having them control us. This practice gives kids a way to notice what story they are telling themselves about future or past events, and to reflect on whether what they think is actually true.

You might like to reinforce the concept that having thoughts is normal, and that we are not asking them NOT to have thoughts. Instead, we are practicing the difficult skill of noticing our thoughts and then choosing to let them go or redirect them if we want to.

Introduction

Say: *Today we're going to try a different mindfulness practice. This time we are going to try to focus our attention on counting our breaths. Sounds easy, right? But it's actually kind of hard. Let's try it right now. Just close your eyes or look down and try to count 5 breaths.*

Pause

How did you do? Did your mind wander away and start thinking about something else? Maybe you noticed you were hungry or maybe you were thinking "this is weird!" or maybe you were wondering if you were the only one sitting here with your eyes closed. What did you notice?

Take a few answers.

Say: *One thing we probably all notice is that our minds wander. The good news is that this is perfectly normal. It happens to everyone.*

The difference is that when your mind wanders when you are in math class you might not notice it until the teacher calls on you and you suddenly realize you have no idea what is going on. That's not a great feeling.

Mindfulness helps us notice that moment when our minds wander and see where our minds go. Then we can decide if we want to redirect our minds. That's part of the fun. The ability to notice what is happening in our own minds is called metacognition. We'll be talking a lot about metacognition in Peace of Mind class this year.

It's sort of like you have a remote control in your mind. You might have decided to watch the "Listen to the teacher channel" or the "Do your math homework channel" but your mind might take the remote and change it to the "Think about unicorns channel" or the "What's for dinner? channel." This can happen when we are doing mindfulness too.

Today we are going to try to turn our remotes to the "Counting our Breaths Channel." Now this might not be the most exciting channel so we need to help it a bit.

Try to get really curious about what breathing is like. What does it feel like? What is a whole breath? Where do you feel each part of your breath in your body? Do you feel it in your stomach, or chest or nose or throat? This curiosity might make it a little easier to keep your mind on this channel.

Our minds really like to change the channel so as soon as you notice that instead of watching the "Counting Your Breaths Channel" your mind has switched to the "I have a basketball game later channel" or the "Why did I say that embarrassing thing in music class yesterday? channel," see if you can take the remote back and reprogram it to the "Count your breaths channel." You might have to change the channel over and over and that is perfectly fine. Trying to get better at this is one of the most useful things we can do!

Mindfulness Practice

Invite today's Mindfulness Leader(s) (ML) to come to the front of the class.

Prompt the ML to say: "Let's sit up a little straighter. Close your eyes or look down into your lap. Let's take 3 deep breaths."

Remote Control Breathing

Say: *Now let your breath settle back into its natural rhythm. Just breathe. Put your hand on your belly to help you to focus on your breath.*

When you are ready, turn your remote control to the "Counting Your Breaths Channel" and start counting your breaths. Then just try to notice if your mind changes the channel and change it back. You might have to do this over and over. That's perfectly fine. Whenever you notice that your mind has changed the channel you might make a little gesture like you are changing the channel back.

Wait about a minute or so (or longer if it seems like they are able to do more) **and then say**: *Now you can just let your mind be free to think or not think.*

After a moment say: *Now take a nice deep breath.*

Optional: Ask the ML to ring the bell.

Say: Open your eyes or look up when you are ready.

Ask the ML to return to their seat(s).

Reflect and Discuss

Remote Control worksheet

Hand out Remote Control worksheets. Have students list any thoughts or feelings they remember having. This activity can also be done in their journals.

Discuss:

- Did your mind change the channel a lot or a little today?
- Was it tempting to stay on a different channel?
- Was it easy or hard to change the channel back?
- When could it be useful to redirect your focus?
- Is there something that you notice yourself thinking about all the time? Are you happy about this or is it something you would like to change?
- **Ask:** Would anyone like to share some of the channels you listed on your worksheet?

Play the Count to Ten Game as in Lesson 3.

Feel free to add this game and other icebreakers into any lesson. They can be helpful in strengthening a sense of community and adding some fun into otherwise challenging lessons.

Peace Partners

Give students time to share what they did for the Peace Partners.

Do the Peace Partner activity as before.

Assign new Peace Partners. Remind your students that their job is to do at least one kind thing for their Peace Partner this week.

Closing words: Okay, our time is up for today. Thank you for a great class, everyone.

Optional: *Let's have a nice quiet moment for the bell. If you want to, you can close your eyes, picture your new Peace Partner, and imagine yourself doing something kind for them this week.*

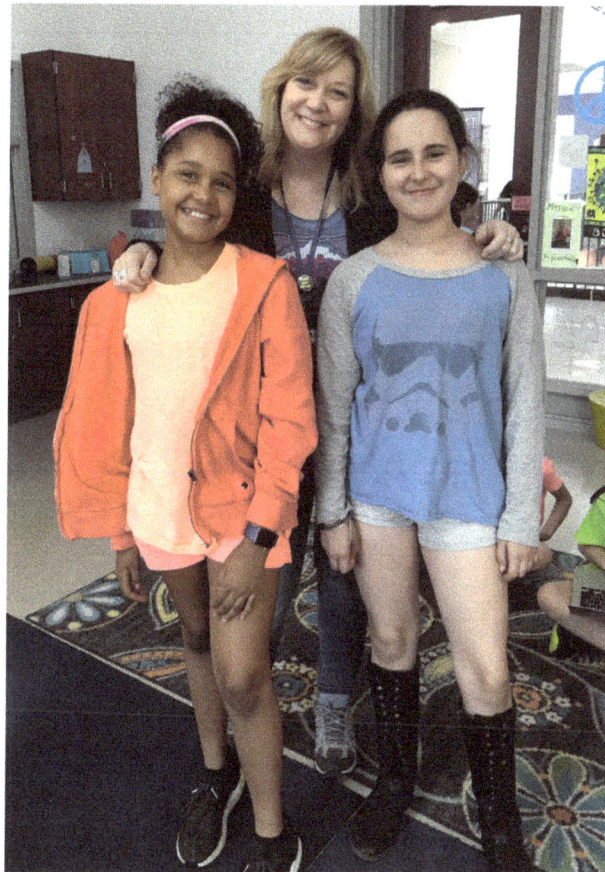

Remote Control Breathing

Your Name _____

Did your mind change the channel during your mindfulness practice?
List some of the channels that you noticed:

_____

_____

_____

_____

_____

_____

_____

_____

_____

_____

_____

_____

_____

UNIT 3
Gratitude and the Negativity Bias

In this unit, we explore our brain's tendency to focus on the negative and how we can balance this tendency with gratitude practice.

Lesson 9
Negativity Bias and the Marble Game

OBJECTIVES: Learn about the Negativity Bias and how we can "hack" our brains to reduce its power

Practice kindness

Assign new Peace Partners

PREPARATION: Review lesson

- Review two Peace of Mind videos: Ms. Ryden explains the Negativity Bias https://www.youtube.com/watch?v=93O7xC0BxVg&feature=youtu.be (starting at minute 7)

- Ms. Ryden reads Sergio Sees the Good. https://www.youtube.com/watch?v=GcwZNzuYjG4&feature=youtu.be

Your Peace Partners list

Enough small cups for every child in your class (if you don't have cups you can just make piles)

Approximately 10 small identical objects for each child (such as marbles or paper clips or whatever you might have). Divide objects into cups so that each *pair* of students may have one cupful.

Optional: Gratitude Box or Jar for the Class/Each Student

Optional: bell or chime

Optional: student journals

The Negativity Bias refers to our brain's tendency to focus on and remember painful, embarrassing, or threatening experiences more than positive ones. The Negativity Bias can be helpful by protecting us from danger. For example, once we've experienced the sting of a bee, we are careful to avoid bees in the future.

But have you ever focused so much on a minor negative experience - being late for a meeting for example - that you've been unable to enjoy the good things going on around you for the rest of the day? If you have (and who hasn't?), you know all about the Negativity Bias.

Today we are going to do an activity that can help students learn how to override the Negativity Bias. They will rewind the day (as in the book *Sergio Sees the Good*) and see if they can remember everything that happened. Our Negativity Bias is focused on helping us remember negative things, but if we make an effort, we can also remember and focus on positive things.

Unless we're in immediate danger, it's possible and more helpful to focus on the positive things in our lives. We'll explore how practicing gratitude can transform our perception of our days.

Recommended reading: Take in the Good by Rick Hanson, Ph.D.

Introduction

Say: *Today we're going to be learning about a characteristic of our brains — the Negativity Bias -- that sometimes makes it harder to remember the good things that happen to us.*

We're also going to be talking about gratitude. Gratitude is the feeling of being thankful. We can be thankful, or grateful, for all kinds of things and people and food and nature. We'll find out about the relationship between the Negativity Bias and gratitude.

We're going to start out by thinking of what we are grateful for and then we're going to do a little mindfulness practice to help us feel gratitude.

Mindfulness Practice

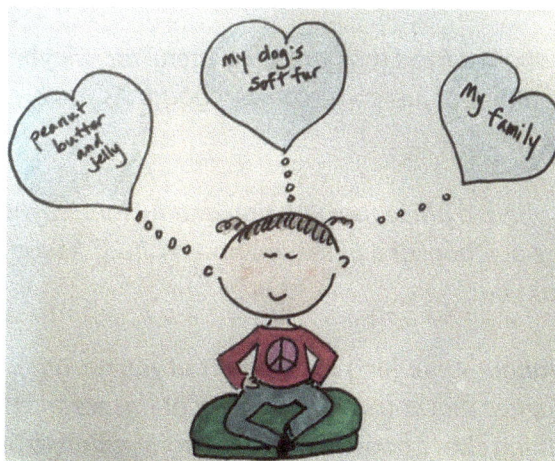

Say: *Today we are going to try a new mindfulness practice that focuses on gratitude. Gratitude is the practice of noticing what we are thankful for, and expressing our thanks.*

We are going to be creating a web of gratitude.

Later in class we are going to be writing about what we placed in our web of gratitude. If you want to you can imagine this picture while you do the practice. (Optional: Show the picture above.)

We'll be thinking about people or things that we are grateful for and we'll be imagining that we are putting them in our web of gratitude. You can imagine your web anyway that you want.

Think about a visual that helps you to see how you are connected to all of the people and things in your web of gratitude.

Invite today's Mindful Leader(s) (ML) to come to the front of the class.

Prompt the ML to say: "Let's sit up a little straighter. Close your eyes or look down into your lap. Let's take 3 deep breaths."

Say: *Let's start by thinking about a **person** that you are thankful, or grateful for. Think of someone who helps you and is kind to you. Imagine that they are in one of the little hearts in your web of gratitude. As you breathe in and out think "Thank you."*

*Next, let's think about a **thing**, an object, that you are grateful for. Why is it important to you? What does it mean to you? As you breathe in and out think "Thank you."*

*Now let's think about a **food** that you are grateful for. Maybe it is a favorite dish from your culture, or just some comfort good. As you breathe in and out think "Thank you."*

*Now let's think about a **place** that you are grateful for. Maybe it's a park or somewhere here at school or a place you have visited. As you breathe in and out think "Thank you."*

*Now let's think about something in **nature** that you are grateful for. Maybe there is a special tree that you love or a flower or the ocean or the moon or snow, or something else. Choose something from nature to put into your web of gratitude. As you breathe in, and out think "Thank you."*

*Now this time you can think about **anyone or anything** that you are feeling grateful to have in your life. Imagine adding that person or thing to your web of gratitude. As you breathe in and out think "Thank you."*

Add on any other gratitude focus that you think might be helpful to your class.

Take a moment to soak in this feeling of gratitude. Notice what it feels like in your body to be grateful and to say thank you. Remember that you can do this practice on your own anytime.

Let's take a deep breath in and stretch your arms up over your head and then slowly float your arms down as you breathe out.

Say: *Take a moment to notice how you feel. Any way that you feel is fine, even if you feel nothing. Just try to notice it.*

Optional: Ask ML to ring the bell.

Ask students to open their eyes and/or look up when they are ready.

Cue the ML to return to their seat(s).

Discuss

- What was that like for you?
- Would anyone like to share anything in their web of gratitude?

The Negativity Bias

Introduce the Negativity Bias

Say: *If we touch a cactus and get hurt, our brain will file that memory in order to prevent us from doing it again. That's helpful. Scientists call this the Negativity Bias. This means that our brains tend to focus on and remember negative things more than positive things. This is one way our brain works to protect us.*

Most of the time, though, it would help us to focus more on the positive events in our lives. Of course, we remember the big good things like our birthday, or a great trip, or a special event. But we often forget all about small good things.

Scientists have found that a great way to balance out our brain's tendency to focus on negative things is to take a moment to consciously soak in positive things.

Taking time to notice and really focus on something good that happens allows our brains to send those memories to long-term storage and helps to train our brain to focus on the positive more often.

Focusing on the positive doesn't mean that we are trying to avoid negative things. Not at all. Our brains will take care of that for us. By helping our brains recognize and soak in positive things, we are helping our brains to see our lives more realistically.

Sergio's Scales Activity

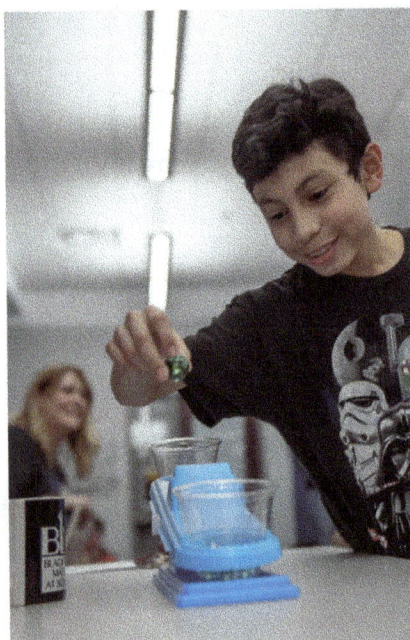

It would be possible to review our days individually, deciding what was good and what was bad on our own. But there is a particular power in doing this activity in pairs. Having someone else listen closely and then mark the good and the bad for us helps us feel truly heard. This exercise when done in pairs can help to build deeper connections among students in your class.

Say: *Today you are going to work with your Peace Partner to do an activity that can help you to override the Negativity Bias. You're going to try to rewind your day, or yesterday, and see if you can remember everything that happened.*

Our Negativity Bias is focused on helping you remember negative things, but if we make an effort to remember and focus on positive things it can help to balance the scales a bit.

Ask a volunteer to hand out two empty cups and one cup full of objects to each pair. **Have** the students label their empty cups "good" and "bad."

Directions

- Decide who will go first.

- The person who goes first will remember out loud everything about their day from the time they woke up. You can decide what you want to share - it doesn't have to be everything.

- As the first person talks, their partner will put objects in either the "good" or "bad" cup for each event.

- When you have reached the present moment, take a minute to notice: has the day been more good or bad so far?

- When the first person has finished, return the objects to their starting cup.

- The other person takes their turn.

- Important: students may not choose to share every event in their day so far, and that is fine. As in all of our lessons, please respect students' decisions about how much to participate and share.

Reflect and Discuss

- Who was surprised by what you found?

- What were some of the good things you noticed?

- Did you notice that you had forgotten a lot of little good things?

- How did it feel to have your partner listening to you and putting marbles in cups for you?

Gratitude Practice

Consider introducing a way for your class to keep track of what they are grateful for. This might include:

- Creating personal Gratitude Jars, Boxes or using their Journals and adding something each week.

- Creating a class Gratitude Jar or Box and adding something each week.

Peace Partners

Give students time to share what they did for the Peace Partners.

Optional: Tell your partner one thing you are grateful for, write it down and put it in the Gratitude Box.

Assign new Peace Partners. Remind your students that their job is to do at least one kind thing for their Peace Partner this week.

Closing words: *Okay, our time is up for today. Thank you for a great class, everyone.*

Optional: *Let's have a nice quiet moment for the bell. If you want to, you can close your eyes, picture your new Peace Partner, and imagine yourself doing something kind for them this week.*

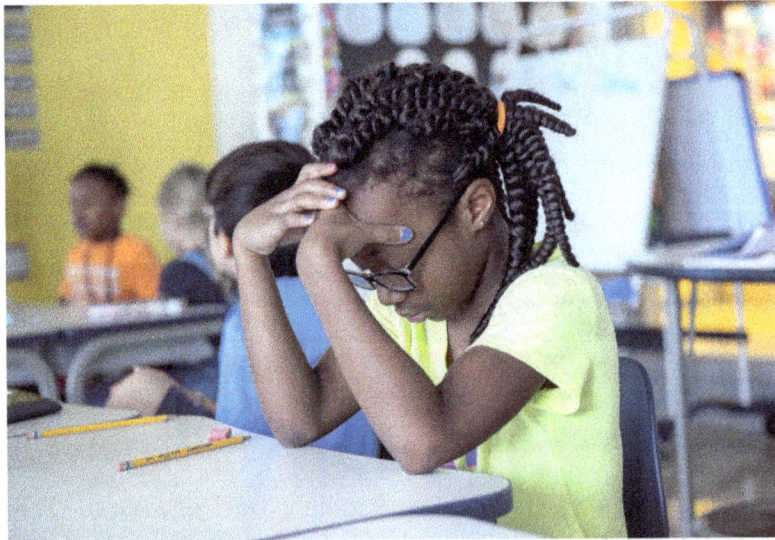

Lesson 10
Expressing Gratitude

OBJECTIVES:
Practice gratitude

Recognize how expressing gratitude makes you feel

Practice kindness

Assign new Peace Partners

PREPARATION:
Review lesson

Your Peace Partners list

Prepare to show the video What Teens Are Thankful For https://www.youtube.com/watch?v=aqLXGiqT2ZE

Index cards with names/photos of all school staff

Materials for making gratitude cards: white paper, markers

Optional: bell or chime

Optional: student journals

In the last lesson, we experienced the power of gratitude practice to balance out our brain's Negativity Bias. In this lesson, we explore another way expressing gratitude increases our well-being. The video from the Greater Good Science Center is about the power of not just feeling, but also expressing, gratitude. (For more practices like this one, visit Greater Good in Education at www.ggie.berkeley.edu and Mindful Schools at www.mindfulschools.org.) Students will then have a chance to express gratitude to school staff by making thank you cards. If possible, students might personally deliver and read their cards to the staff members.

Introduction

You might say: *Today we are going to be saying thank you to some important people in our lives right in our school building. I know that many of you have made birthday cards for your family members or friends.*

But have you ever said thank you to our custodians? Or the front-office staff? Or the dedicated people who make our lunches in the cafeteria? Well, here's your chance!

Today we are going to show our thanks to the important people who keep our school running. I'm going to ask you to choose somebody at our school that you want to thank and make that person a thank you card to express our gratitude for all of their hard work. Try to think of someone who might not usually get thanks.

Say: *As always, we'll begin with mindfulness practice to help us get ready.*

Mindfulness Practice

Invite today's Mindful Leader(s) (ML) to come to the front of the class.

Prompt the ML to say: "Let's sit up a little straighter. Close your eyes or look down into your lap. Let's take 3 deep breaths."

Say: *So let's begin:*

*Let's start by thinking about a **person** that you are thankful, or grateful for. Think of someone who helps you and is kind to you. Imagine that they are in one of the little hearts in your web of gratitude. As you breathe in and out think "Thank you."*

*Next, let's think about a **thing**, an object, that you are grateful for. Why is it important to you? What does it mean to you? As you breathe in and out think "Thank you."*

*Now let's think about a **food** that you are grateful for. Maybe it is a favorite dish from your culture, or just some comfort good. As you breathe in and out think "Thank you."*

*Now let's think about a **place** that you are grateful for. Maybe it's a park or somewhere here at school or a place you have visited. As you breathe in and out think "Thank you."*

*Now let's think about something in **nature** that you are grateful for. Maybe there is a special tree that you love or a flower or the ocean or the moon or snow, or something else. Choose something from nature to put into your web of gratitude. As you breathe in, and out think "Thank you."*

*Now this time you can think about **anyone or anything** that you are feeling grateful to have in your life. Imagine adding that person or thing to your web of gratitude. As you breathe in and out think "Thank you."*

Take a moment to soak in this feeling of gratitude. Notice what it feels like in your body to be grateful and to say thank you. Remember that you can do this practice on your own anytime.

Add on any other gratitude focus that you think might be helpful to your class.

Say*: Let's take a deep breath in and stretch your arms up over your head and then slowly float your arms down as you breathe out.*

Optional: Ask ML to ring the bell.

Ask students to open their eyes and/or look up when they are ready.

Cue the ML to return to their seat(s).

Ask: What was that like for you?

Take a few answers.

What Teens are Thankful For

Watch this video <u>What Teens Are Thankful For</u>. https://www.youtube.com/watch?v=aqLXGiqT2ZE

Ask: Who are the people in your lives for whom you are grateful?

Gratitude Practice

Ask a volunteer to help distribute supplies: paper and crayons and markers.

Give out index cards with names of every member of your school's staff. If possible, include pictures of each person.

Invite students to make a card expressing gratitude for the person on their card.

Collect the cards when students are finished.

If possible, have the students hand-deliver or even read the cards to their recipients.

Peace Partners

Give students time to share what they did for the Peace Partners.

Do the Peace Partner activity as before.

Assign new Peace Partners. Remind your students that their job is to do at least one kind thing for their Peace Partner this week.

Closing words: *Okay, our time is up for today. Thank you for a great class, everyone.*

Optional*: Let's have a nice quiet moment for the bell. If you want to, you can close your eyes, picture your new Peace Partner, and imagine yourself doing something kind for them this week.*

UNIT 4
Your Brain and Your Thoughts

In this unit, we review the functions and interrelatedness of three key parts of our brains: the amygdala, the hippo-campus and the prefrontal cortex. We put this knowledge to work in role plays and skits.

Lesson 11
Where Are My Thoughts?

Objectives: Notice if thoughts are mostly about the past, present or future

Continue to learn about metacognition

Practice kindness

Assign new Peace Partners

Preparation: Review lesson

Your Peace Partners list

Optional: bell or chime

Optional: student journals

The object of this lesson is to help students learn that they have the choice of focusing on the present moment. This is another way to use the skill of meta-cognition. Students will learn how to direct their thoughts away from worries about the past or future, to notice when they are thinking about imaginary scenarios, and to stay in the present moment.

Some of us are prone to worry and rumination. This practice offers a way to use mindful breathing to notice, allow and then manage this way of responding to challenging situations. This practice also gives students a way to manage their reactions to emotions inspired by others – to stay in control of their own responses.

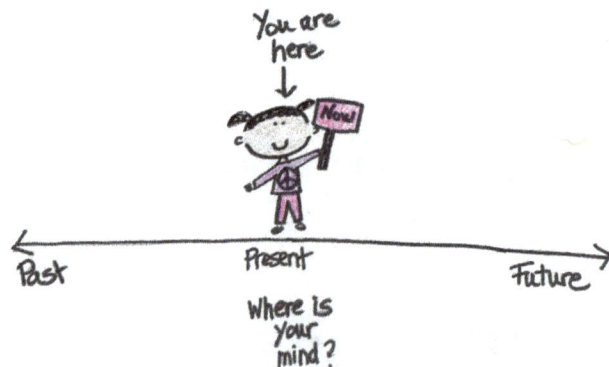

Introduction

You might say:

A few lessons ago, we practiced noticing our thoughts. We imagined that we had a remote control in our minds and noticed what channel we were on. Today we are going to do something similar. We are going to try to notice if our thoughts are about the past, the present, or the future.

We might imagine that remote control again but this time there are only a few channels. You might think of them as The History Channel (the past), the Sci-Fi Channel (the future) and The Right Now Channel (the present). This is actually a very challenging practice.

If I am thinking about my basketball game tomorrow my thoughts are in the... (**future**). The Sci-Fi Channel

If I am thinking about an argument I had with my little brother last night, my thoughts are in the… (**past**). The History Channel

if I am noticing that I am hungry my thoughts are in the … (**present**). The Right Now Channel

Sometimes you might notice that your thoughts aren't about the past, present or future but are just imaginings - maybe you are thinking about riding on a unicorn. That isn't something that you did in the past or will do in the future but just a different kind of thought.

What would be a good name for that channel? The Imagination Channel? The Anything Goes Channel?

Have them make their own names

Say: Last time whenever we noticed that our minds had changed the channel we made a little changing channels gesture with our hands. Let's make up some new gestures for this game.

One way to do this is to say your left hand is for the past, your right hand is for the future and both hands in the middle is for the present. If you notice a past thought you could raise your left hand, if you notice a future thought you could raise your right hand, if you notice a present thought you can bring your hands together for a present thought.

Who can think of a gesture that would show that you were having an imaginary thought?

Take some ideas and let kids choose their own as long as they aren't distracting to others.

Demonstrate this for your students by narrating your own thoughts, labeling each one as in the past, present, future or imagination. If students ask questions about imaginary thoughts vs. future thoughts, you can let them know it doesn't really matter what they call the thoughts, but it is important to notice them and to try to let them go to come back to the present moment.

Say: *So today, after we get set up by the Mindfulness Leader, we are going to try to count our breaths.*

Only this time, every time you notice that your mind has wandered (and you know it will!) I want you to try to notice if it is a thought about the past, the present, the future, or an imaginary thought.

Once you've labeled that thought, see if you can bring your mind back to counting your breaths.

Mindfulness Practice

Invite today's Mindfulness Leader(s) (ML) to come to the front of the class.

Prompt the ML to say: "Let's sit up a little straighter. Close your eyes or look down into your lap. Let's take 3 deep breaths."

Lead the class through Past-Present-Future as described above.

You might say: *Continue breathing in and out.*

When you notice that your focus has wandered away from your breathing, notice if you are thinking about something that happened in the past or the future, or whether it is about something that is happening right now.

Bring your mind back to your breathing. You might want to try counting your breaths to help you.

After a few moments, say: *Now take one more deep breath in and out.*

Optional: Ask ML to ring the bell.

Ask students to open their eyes and/or look up when they are ready.

Cue the ML to return to their seat(s).

- Where were your thoughts?
- Raise your hand if most of your thoughts were about the past.
- Raise your hand if most of your thoughts were in the present.
- Raise your hand if most of your thoughts were in the future.
- Raise your hand if most of your thoughts were imaginary.
- Raise your hand if you had a mixture.

Ask some of the students to share one of the thoughts they noticed and then let other students guess if the thought was in the past, present, or future. This isn't always easy and there can be more than one right answer.

Discuss:

- Why do you think it might be good to keep your mind focused on the present, on this moment?
- If your mind is always focused on what has already happened, or what hasn't happened yet, or what might never happen, what do you think you might be missing?

Point out:

- When we try to notice where our thoughts are going, we can try to redirect them to where we want them to be. If you tend to worry a lot, your thoughts are mostly in the.. (future).
- Worrying doesn't help make things better and it doesn't stop bad things from happening. But it does keep you from enjoying the good stuff.
- If you notice that your thoughts are often in the future, see if you can try to focus your mind on something right here in the present moment. Try to notice what is good in this moment.
- Perhaps share an example from your own life of the value of focusing on the present moment, instead of on the past or future.

Written Reflection

Using the worksheet from Week 8, or student Journals, invite students to record their thoughts, dividing them into past, present, future and imagination.

Ask them to notice what surprises them, or whether they gain any insights from noticing the pattern of their thoughts.

Peace Partners

Give students time to share what they did for the Peace Partners.

Do the Peace Partner activity as before.

Assign new Peace Partners. Remind your students that their job is to do at least one kind thing for their Peace Partner this week.

Closing words: *Okay, our time is up for today. Thank you for a great class, everyone.*

Optional: *Let's have a nice quiet moment for the bell. If you want to, you can close your eyes, picture your new Peace Partner, and imagine yourself doing something kind for them this week.*

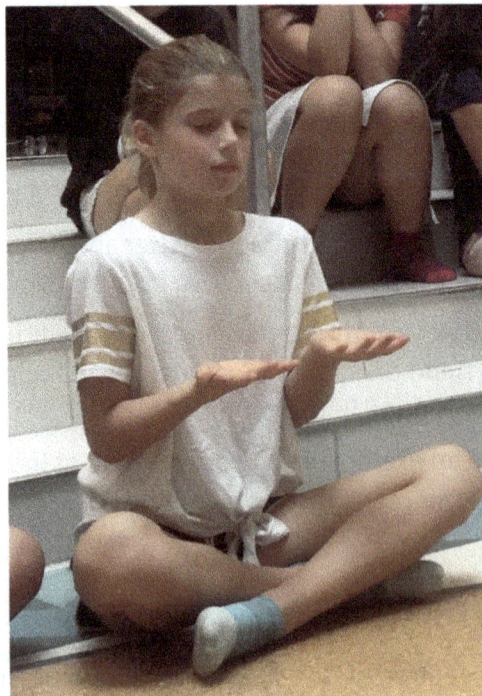

Lesson 12
Meet Your Brain

Objectives:	**Familiarize students with three key parts of the brain**
	Practice kindness
	Assign new Peace Partners
Preparation:	**Review lesson**
	Post Brain Poster in a visible place (at end of lesson).
	Watch Dr. Dan Siegel's video as background : **https://www.YouTube.com/watch?v=f-m2YcdMdFw**
	Watch Peace of Mind's Take Five Breathing video **https://www.youtube.com/watch?v=BSR4a-dRxic&feature=youtu.beto help teach this practice**
	Prepare to show this video Fight Flight Freeze – Anxiety Explained For Teens https://www.youtube.com/watch?v=rpolpKTWrp4
	Optional: bell or chime
	Optional: Student Journal

Our brains are complex and quite amazing parts of our bodies. In this curriculum, we offer a simplified look at how our brains work in order to help students' understand why we practice mindfulness and how it helps. We focus on two important components of the limbic system, the amygdala and the hippocampus, and also on the integrating portion of the brain's cortex, the prefrontal cortex.

By giving students insight into how their brains work, we help them realize that they have the ability to control how they respond to stimuli.

Introduction

You might say: *Today we're going to be learning a little bit about our brains. And then we'll learn a new mindfulness practice called Take Five Breathing. Today we're going to do the mindfulness practice a little later in the lesson.*

Learning about our brains can help us to understand why we do the things we do. Let's start out by thinking about anger.

Can you think of some times when you got angry? Maybe you were supposed to go to a party and then your parents told you that you couldn't go because you had to babysit for your little sister. Or you tried out for the basketball team and didn't make it.

Ask them to share some examples.

Then share the scenarios below and have them talk with their Peace Partner about how they would feel and how they would typically react.

Ask them to think about these questions for each scenario. Suggest that students think back to Lesson 7 when we paid attention to where we feel emotions in our bodies. For each scenario, invite students to consider:

1. How would you handle this situation?
2. How does that usually work for you?

You might invite Peace Partners to talk about each emotion together, and then invite students to share out. Or a smaller group might discuss these questions as a group for each scenario.

List answers/emotions on the board.

Scenarios:

- You were invited to a party but you can't go because you have to babysit for your little sister.
- You tried out for the basketball team and didn't make it.
- You're on the basketball team but you're almost always sitting on the bench during games.
- Your friends are all going to a concert but you can't afford the ticket.
- Your best friend got the sneakers you wanted but your parents won't get them for you.
- You see on Instagram that your friend had people over but didn't invite you.
- You auditioned for a solo in the choir concert and didn't get it.
- You finished your Social Studies paper but you left it at home and you're going to be marked down for lateness.

Notice how often students say that their chosen method of resolution works or doesn't work for them.

You might say: *It can help to understand what is happening in your brain when these things happen. We're going to be learning about three parts of the brain. When we know what's happening physiologically, we have a better understanding of how we can manage our big emotions and arrive at solutions to problems that get us where we want to go in a positive way.*

Brain science, or neuroscience is really complicated, even for people who study it all the time. Neuroscientists are constantly learning new things about the brain. We're going to dive into a relatively simple overview. The parts we are going to talk about are really important to understand because knowing about them can help us to understand why we do some of the things we do, especially when we get angry.

Point out Brain Poster and three parts of the brain.

Prefrontal Cortex

*The first part we're going to talk about is the **Prefrontal Cortex or PFC**. (show on poster). The PFC is like the boss of your brain. It makes decisions and choices and helps the other parts to work together. The PFC keeps growing until you are in your mid-twenties. Most of the time your PFC is in charge of your brain. Put your hand on your forehead: your PFC is right behind your skull.*

Hippocampus

Another interesting part of your brain is called the Hippocampus. This is the part of the brain that makes and stores your memories. You might think of the Hippocampus as the librarian of your brain - storing up all of your memories like books in a library or your hard drive. It's deep inside your brain. (show on poster).

Amygdala

The last part we're going to learn about is the Amygdala. The amygdala is one of the most interesting and one of the most troublesome parts of the brain. The amygdala is like your brain's security guard. It is always on the lookout for danger. When the amygdala thinks you're in danger it reacts. It doesn't think, it just reacts. (show on poster).

This might sound weird (or it might not), but you've already experienced this.

Amygdala in action

1. Protection

- Give everyone a piece of paper and ask them to ball it up.
- Have them turn to their partner and take turns gently tossing the ball at each other's head. See what happens to their eyes.
- Prompt them to notice: What are they feeling?
- Prompt them to notice: Do they want to block their face with their hands?

Ask: *So what happened? If someone throws a ball at you what do you do? Maybe you catch it or push it away from you. You don't decide to do those things - you just have a reflex that makes you do it. You DON'T watch the ball calmly as it flies at your head. That reflex is controlled by the Amygdala. It doesn't think it just reacts. That is the Amygdala protecting your face and brain. That's why we blink when something gets near our eyes or flinch when we hear a loud, surprising noise.*

Can you think of examples of when you think your Amygdala was protecting you? Maybe you turn around to see who is coming in when somebody opens the door, maybe you run away when you see a dog that looks dangerous, or you jump back onto the curb when you are crossing the street if you hear a car coming. Your amygdala has probably already saved your life many times.

ASK them to share examples.

2. Anger

But, the amygdala sometimes totally overreacts. Has this ever happened to you? You are playing a video game and someone calls you for dinner. Even though you like eating, and you like whoever called you, you start yelling and making a big fuss.

Maybe somebody accidentally bumps into you and knocks your backpack out of your hands. They are really sorry and try to help you but you can't help but yell at them. Welcome to the down side of the Amygdala!

Let's go back to the scenarios we talked about at the beginning of class. Can you see how the amygdala was protecting you in any of those situations?

It's as if the Amygdala can't tell the difference between a real danger - like getting attacked by a bear- and something that you just don't like - like having to stop your game or dropping your backpack. It reacts the same way. The amygdala doesn't think - it just reacts and that's why it is both a really helpful and really difficult part of the brain.

Sometimes when people have to deal with scary things a lot in their real lives - maybe there is violence in their neighborhood or someone at school is threatening them - their amygdalas are working overtime. They can start to over-react to every little thing. It's almost like their security guard (the amygdala) is on high alert all the time. Always ready to fight. You might know people like this or maybe you feel a little like this yourself.

3. Anxiety

Your amygdala isn't just responsible for anger - but also for other emotions like anxiety. Let's see how this works.

Watch *Fight Flight Freeze – Anxiety Explained For Teens*

Discuss

- How do you know when your amygdala is overreacting?
- Do you think some of the mindful breathing practices we've been learning could be helpful?

Your brain and your body: what do you notice?

You might say: Think about how you feel when you are angry or nervous or scared. What do you notice in your body?

Invite students to share.

Say: *Do you notice anything different about your breathing? You might notice that when you are angry or scared or nervous your breathing is shallow and fast - like panting.*

This is what it feels like when your amygdala takes over your brain - it's getting your body ready to fight or run away. You might feel really out of control when this happens.

And when you're out of control, other people can control you.

Mindfulness Practice: Keeping your power

Say: *One way to help you to keep your power and stay in control of yourself is to do a simple breathing technique. This isn't just to relax you. It can send a message to your amygdala that everything is okay so that you can stop and think about what you want to do. So you are in control again.*

This technique is called **Take Five Breathing.** *To do Take Five, you trace one of your hands with the index finger of the other hand.*

Share the Take Five Breathing video here if you think it would be helpful. https://www.youtube.com/watch?v=BSR4a-dRxic&feature=youtu.be

As you trace up, you take a gentle but deep breath in. When you trace down, you gently breathe out. You will repeat until you have traced all of your fingers.

By this time you have taken five deep breaths and would have possibly convinced your amygdala that everything is okay and that it can stand down and let the PFC take over. That's the part of your brain that can figure out what to do. So, let's try it.

Invite today's Mindfulness Leader (ML) to come to the front of the class.

Prompt the ML to say: "Let's sit up a little straighter. Close your eyes or look down into your lap. Let's take 3 deep breaths."

Say: *Now we'll do some Take Five Breathing. Trace up your thumb and take a deep but gentle breath in. When you trace down gently breathe out. Repeat until you have traced all of your fingers.*

After you have finished tracing your hand, take one more deep breath in and out.

Ask students to open their eyes and/or look up when they are ready.

Cue the ML to return to their seat(s).

Ask: How do you feel?

Take a few answers.

Say: *Today we had our Mindful Leaders(s) get us ready for this practice, and that was great. But notice you can do Take Five - like any of the practices we are learning - anytime. You don't have to be sitting at your desk.*

94 |

Peace Partners

Give students time to share what they did for their Peace Partners.

Do the Peace Partner activity as before.

Assign new Peace Partners. Remind your students that their job is to do at least one kind thing for their Peace Partner this week.

Closing words: *Okay, our time is up for today. Thank you for a great class, everyone.*

Optional: *Let's have a nice quiet moment for the bell. If you want to, you can close your eyes, picture your new Peace Partner, and imagine yourself doing something kind for them this week.*

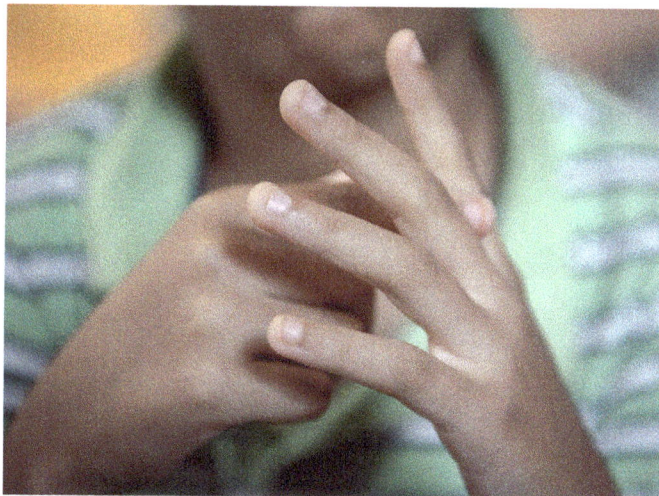

Diagram of Three Parts of the Brain

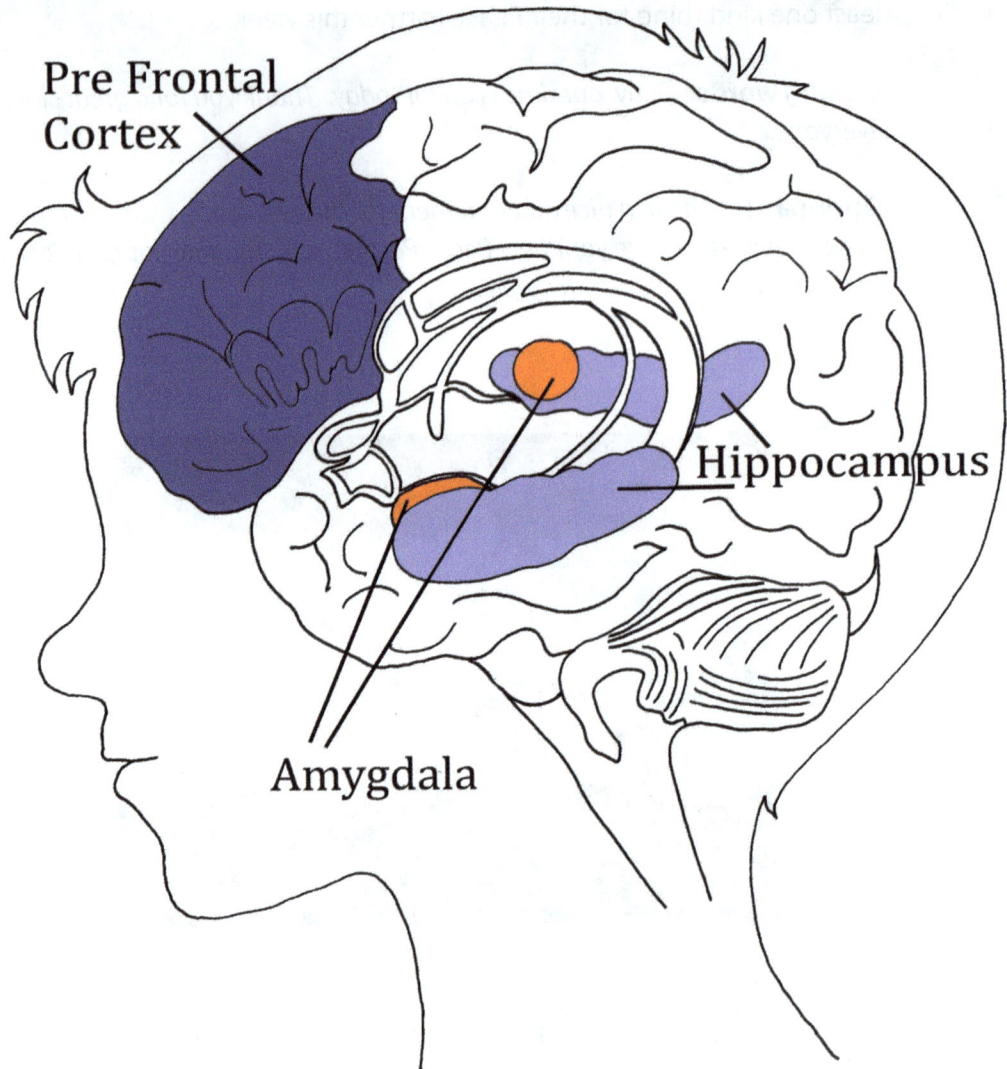

Pre Frontal Cortex

Hippocampus

Amygdala

Lesson 13
Your Brain and Basketball

OBJECTIVES: Review the three parts of the brain with the poster

Choose a mindfulness practice

Deepen understanding of how 3 parts of the brain are interrelated

Practice kindness

Assign new Peace Partners

PREPARATION: Review lesson

Post Brain Poster in a visible place

4 Copies of the *Elijah's Brain* skit found at at end of lesson, if needed

Optional: bell or chime

Optional: student journals

Today we will work on reinforcing the relevance of understanding how our brains work and how and why mindfulness skills can help us keep control of our responses. Kids will have the opportunity to read or act out a skit called Elijah's Brain and make a connection to the Under Pressure video we saw in Lesson 1 - perhaps focusing on the way in which mindfulness helps the featured basketball players.

Introduction

Say: *Today we are going to review the roles of amygdala, hippocampus and prefrontal cortex, and then [**whatever you decide**: read/act out a skit called "Elijah's Brain" and/or reflect creatively on the connection between big emotions, your brain, and mindfulness.]*

But first, we start with our mindfulness practice. Today you can choose from one of the mindfulness practices that we've learned so far. You might want to choose one of the breathing practices that help us to calm down like Take Five, Four Square, and Clench and Release.

It's important to figure out which practice works best for you. Everybody's different and that's why we're learning so many different practices.

Mindfulness Practice

Invite today's Mindfulness Leader (ML) to come to the front of the class.

Prompt the ML to say: "Let's sit up a little straighter. Close your eyes or look down into your lap. Let's take 3 deep breaths."

Invite students to choose a practice like Take Five, Four Square Breathing, or Clench and Release.

After a few moments, say: *Now take one more deep breath in and out.*

Optional: Ask ML to ring the bell.

Ask students to open their eyes and/or look up when they are ready.

Cue the ML to return to their seat(s).

Using brain knowledge to help manage anger

Say: *I am going to share a situation with you and then ask you how you feel.*

Say: *Imagine that you are hanging out with a friend on a Saturday. You have a new video game you really want to play but when your friend arrives they say that they want to go to the park and play soccer.*

Ask the class:

- How do you feel? (Angry, upset, disappointed?)
- What does your amygdala tell you to do? (Get angry, yell, tell them that if you can't play your game you don't want to hang out with them, keep your feelings to yourself but still feel angry, some other way....)
- How will things turn out if you only listen to your amygdala? (Your friend will be mad, you will miss out, they might go home, won't want to hang out with you anymore…)

Say: *Have you ever heard the term "flipping your lid?" Dr. Dan Siegel uses it to explain what happens in our brains when we get angry.*

We can use our hand to be a model of the brain. Make a fist with your thumb tucked in. When your fist is closed you are calm. Your amygdala is keeping watch and your Prefrontal Cortex (your knuckles) is in charge and making decisions. The hippocampus (on the palm inside your fist) can access memories. But when we get angry, we "flip our lid."

Flip your fingers up exposing the amygdala.

It can feel like our amygdala is in charge, and we can't think very well because our Prefrontal Cortex or PFC is no longer in charge. You really need your Prefrontal Cortex (or PFC) to help you work this out. But how can you get it back in charge again?

When we take our deep breaths and take care of our anger, it helps to bring our Prefrontal Cortex back in charge.

Fold your fingers down slowly.

It can take a little while to work, but once we have our lids back on we can think about what we want to do. We have choices.

Putting the PFC Back In Charge

Once you have your lid back on and your PFC is in charge, you can think about how much you like your friend, and you start to think about your options.

Ask: *What are some other ways to solve this problem? (Take turns playing soccer and video games, let your guest decide what to play, and so on.)*

Say: *Do you see how your PFC helps you see that you have choices and sometimes what your amygdala wants you to do isn't always the best idea?*

The next time you get angry, see if you can remember that this is your amygdala talking to you. See if you can use your breathing to help take care of your amygdala.

It's important to remember that your amygdala is trying to take care of you. If you feel angry or upset that is fine. All of your emotions are fine.

The problem with anger is that sometimes the way we express it can make things worse for us and for those around us.

Once you have calmed down, you can figure out the best way to express what is bothering you so that you can take care of it.

We are not trying to get rid of our anger or any of our emotions. We're just trying to make sure that our feelings aren't controlling us.

Anger, Your Brain and Mindfulness

Here are three options to help students explore the connection between big emotions like anger, their brains, and mindfulness.

1. Assign roles and act out the *Elijah's Brain* skit.
2. Assign roles and have students read the skit from their seats.
3. Reflection in writing or another creative form

Options 1 and 2: Act out or read through *Elijah's Brain*

Invite 4 volunteers to participate and assign them roles: Elijah, his amygdala, his hippocampus, and his prefrontal cortex.

Pass out scripts and have the students act out or read through the skit.

Invite the audience to notice what they feel in their bodies as they watch or listen to the skit.

Discuss:

- Why did Elijah's amygdala decide to take over?
- What was the amygdala's plan for Elijah?
- How would things have turned out if Elijah had let his amygdala take over?
- Why did the amygdala suggest that Elijah either stand still, throw the ball hard, or run away? (the fight, flight or freeze reflex)
- How did the hippocampus and PFC help Elijah to make the shot?
- What kinds of things might be upsetting or distracting during a basketball game?
- The video *Under Pressure* featured a lot of famous basketball players who practice mindfulness. How do you think mindfulness might help them play better?

- How could mindfulness and what you know about your brain help you play better?

Option 3: Reflection

Ask students to reflect on the following questions. This project could take the shape of an essay, a comic, a storyboard, or something else.

- Write about a time you got angry.
- Did your brain choose fight, flight or freeze?
- How did that work out?
- What could your PFC have helped you to choose instead?

Mindful Challenge Game

To introduce the game, say: *Remember the Walk Stop Wiggle Game from Lesson 5? This is actually a brain game that challenges another part of our brains, the prefrontal cortex, to focus on one thing intently, ignoring distractions.*

Let's see if you've gotten any better at this game.

Directions

- There are many levels of this game. In each level, see if you can follow my directions.
- We're going to play the game silently so that everyone can hear the directions.
- Make sure that you are not talking and that you are not touching each other.

Level 1: When I say walk, you walk. When I say stop, you stop. When I say wiggle, you wiggle. When I say sit, you sit. Got it?

> `Level 2:   This time Walk = Stop
>   Stop = Walk
>   Wiggle = Wiggle
>   Sit = Sit

> Level 3:   Walk = Stop
>   Stop = Walk

Wiggle = Sit
Sit = Wiggle

Level 4:   Walk = Wiggle
Wiggle = Walk
Sit = Stop
Stop = Sit

You can keep going, changing up the commands or add in new ones. It's pretty hard!

Peace Partners

Give students time to share what they did for the Peace Partners.

Do the Peace Partner activity as before.

Assign new Peace Partners. Remind your students that their job is to do at least one kind thing for their Peace Partner this week.

Closing words: *Okay, our time is up for today. Thank you for a great class, everyone.*

Optional: *Let's have a nice quiet moment for the bell. If you want to, you can close your eyes, picture your new Peace Partner, and imagine yourself doing something kind for them this week.*

102 | | https://TeachPeaceofMind.org

Elijah's Brain Skit

Topic:	Brain Science
4 Characters:	Elijah, PFC, Amygdala, Hippocampus (Hippo)
Prepare:	Make signs for the brain parts
Setting:	School basketball game. Elijah is preparing to shoot a free throw. His amygdala, PFC and hippocampus are shouting at him from the stands.

PFC: Okay Elijah, you got this. Stay calm and focus on making the shot.

Hippo: Remember what the coach said, aim for the backboard.

Amygdala: Oh no, what if he misses? He's starting to sweat!

PFC: No, it's okay Elijah, just breathe and focus.

Hippo: Remember to bend your knees when you shoot.

Amygdala: No, this is terrible! He's going to miss and then everybody is going to be disappointed and we're going to lose the game!

And hey isn't that Manuel? He's going to make fun of you if you miss.

I'm freaking out!

PFC: Wait, Elijah…

Amygdala: That's enough PFC - I'm going to turn you off!

PFC: Noooooo!!!

Hippo: But Elijah, don't forget…

Amygdala: You too, Hippocampus, off you go. I have a plan. He's going to stand here frozen and then if that doesn't work he can throw the ball really hard and run out of the gym. Perfect!

Hippo: That's terrible advice! Amygdala is just trying to help you but you need to think.

PFC: Do your Take Five breathing!

Elijah starts to do Take Five breathing, tracing one hand with a finger of the other hand, breathing in as he goes up, and out as he goes down.

Amygdala: Wait, what's he doing? Deep breathing? But that means I don't have to be in charge anymore….

PFC: All right! Okay Elijah you got this. Focus!

Hippo: Don't forget to bend your knees Elijah!!

Elijah makes the shot. Everybody cheers!

The End

Lesson 14
Flow

OBJECTIVES:	Learn about the concept of flow
	Learn how flow applies to students' lives
	Practice a new mindfulness exercise
	Practice kindness
	Assign new Peace Partners
PREPARATION:	Review lesson
	Prepare to watch this video on Flow. <u>What is Flow Theory? What does this mean for our students?</u> https://www.youtube.com/watch?v=iUsOCR1KKms(Stop at 2:37).
	Optional: bell or chime
	Optional: student journals

Today we introduce a new Mindfulness concept called "Flow." This concept, coined by psychologist Mihaly Csikszentmihalyi, refers to a state of complete and effortless absorption in the current moment. Flow is also known as being "in the zone" and is often connected to enhanced performance in sports and the arts.

We will watch part of a short video titled "What is Flow Theory?" by John Spencer, Professor, Author and Maker. (For more of Dr. Spencer's work, please visit http//bitly/spencervideos). Then we'll discuss what it feels like for students to be in "the zone," and in what activities they would want to practice flow.

We'll do a mindfulness practice designed to practice getting into the flow state called "more signal, less noise." This practice integrates the skills of attention and mindfulness with maintaining concentration.

Introduction

Say: *Today we are going to explore the concept of flow and apply it to our lives. Flow is another word for being "in the zone." We experience flow when we are fully absorbed in an activity, like a sport, music, or dance. Maybe you have* experienced a feeling of "flow" during a sports game, a music or dance recital, cuddling a pet, or writing a poem.

Watch: What is Flow Theory? What does this mean for our students? (end at 2:37).

Say: *Soon, we will do a mindfulness practice which will let us get into a state of flow more easily. We will do so by calling upon a time when we were completely absorbed in something we were doing and recreating that moment in our minds.*

Take a few moments to think if there is a time where you were "in the zone," or in a state of flow.

Have students share with their neighbor and then take some answers.

Mindfulness Practice

Invite today's Mindful Leader(s) (ML) to come to the front of the class.

Prompt the ML to say: "Let's sit up a little straighter. Close your eyes or look down into your lap. Let's take 3 deep breaths."

Say: *In this mindfulness practice, we are going to explore the experience of flow. Flow is about your body and mind being in the present moment. Let's get a sense of what this feels like.*

First, in your head, ask yourself this question: "Where am I?" Just notice that you are sitting here in this room. Take a second to open your eyes, look straight ahead, but also open up your vision to the sides, or peripheries. If you get distracted, just ask yourself again, "Where am I?"

Now, let's take a moment to feel your body. Feel it sitting, notice the clothes on your body. Notice your breath happening naturally, letting yourself inhale and exhale without effort. The breath is the natural source of flow in our bodies.

Wait about five seconds

Call to mind your unique moment of being "in the zone." This practice will be a visualization, but also a "feeling-ization," because we are going to try to go back and feel, to embody, what our bodies and minds felt like during our experience. Try to imagine all aspects of this moment.

In this moment of flow, where are you?

Wait about five seconds

How does your body feel?

Wait about five seconds

Notice how in this moment you were in a flow state. How in this moment, you weren't worrying or thinking, or straining for a result. Flow is less doing, more existing. When distractions come and take us out of flow, just bring your flow moment to mind and ask yourself, "Where am I?", "How does my body feel?" to come back to the feeling of the flow of your breath and refresh the image and feeling of your flow moment.

After a few moments, say*: Now take one more deep breath in and out.*

Optional: Ask ML to ring the bell.

Ask students to open their eyes and/or look up when they are ready.

Cue the ML to return to their seat(s).

Discuss

- What did this feel like?
- How do you think this practice could be useful to you?

Peace Partners

Give students time to share what they did for the Peace Partners.

Do the Peace Partner activity as before.

Assign new Peace Partners. Remind your students that their job is to do at least one kind thing for their Peace Partner this week.

Give Peace Partners time to share their experiences with Flow today.

Closing words: *Okay, our time is up for today. Thank you for a great class, everyone.*

Optional: *Let's have a nice quiet moment for the bell. If you want to, you can close your eyes, picture your new Peace Partner, and imagine yourself doing something kind for them this week.*

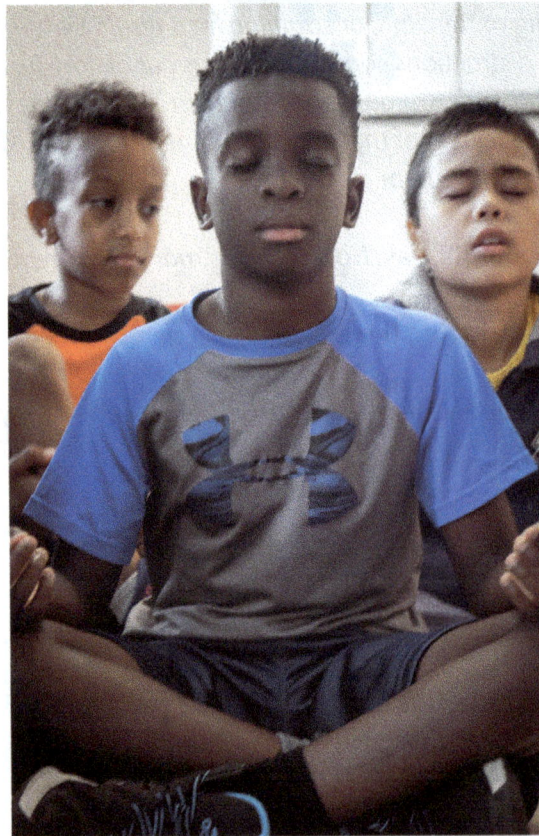

UNIT 5
Conflict Resolution

In this unit, we introduce the concept of the Conflict Escalator, explore what makes a good apology, and meet the Conflict CAT, a method for resolving conflicts. Through discussion, skits and games, we apply what we've been learning about mindfulness, kindness, empathy, and brain science to the challenge of resolving conflicts peacefully.

Going Up the Conflict Escalator

OBJECTIVES:
Learn about what causes conflicts to escalate

Learn a new way to talk about conflict escalation

Use role plays to notice when a conflict is escalating

Engage students in mindfulness

Practice kindness

Assign new Peace Partners

PREPARATION:
Review lesson

Your Peace Partners list

List of conflict scenarios

Two small magnets or post-it notes

Draw the Conflict Escalator on the board

Peace of Mind Gravity Hands Video. https://youtu.be/FfN8KslJqUs

Optional: bell or chime

Optional: student journals

In this lesson we are going to learn about what makes conflict escalate and learn about a way to talk about it - the Conflict Escalator. The Conflict Escalator makes it easier to see what causes a conflict to escalate and then to see how to go about de-escalating. Ideally, when we combine mindfulness skills, an understanding of neuroscience, and some simple conflict resolution skills we can work to not only de-escalate conflicts but learn to prevent them from escalating in the first place, thereby reducing violence in our schools and communities. We're also going to repeat the mindfulness practice See, Hear, Feel from Lesson 5.

Introduction

Say: *Have you ever wondered why you find yourself in an argument when you didn't really mean to be in one? Today we're going to be talking about conflict and something called The Conflict Escalator that helps us understand why*

conflicts that start really small can grow into something that can feel over-whelming. But first, let's do our mindfulness practice. Today we're going to do a new practice called Gravity Hands.

Mindfulness Practice

Say: *Today we're going to learn one more quick mindfulness practice you can use to help you calm down. We call it Gravity Hands.*

To do Gravity Hands, you start with your hands on your knees with your palms facing up. As you slowly breathe in, lift your hands up just about to shoulder height and then slowly turn them over and lower them as you breathe slowly out.

We call this Gravity Hands because you are lifting your hands so slowly that you might feel the gravity of the earth pulling them back down. As you are lowering your hands, you want to resist gravity and bring them slowly down. This slow hand movement can help you to think about breathing very slowly.

Share this Peace of Mind Video of Gravity Hands if it would be helpful.
https://youtu.be/FfN8KslJqUs

Invite today's Mindfulness Leader(s) (ML) to come to the front of the class.

Prompt the ML to say: "Let's sit up a little straighter. Close your eyes or look down into your lap. Let's take some deep breaths."

Say: Let's try Gravity Hands today. Let's take 4-5 deep breaths.

After a few moments, say: *Now take one more deep breath in and out.*

Optional: Ask ML to ring the bell.

Ask students to open their eyes and/or look up when they are ready.

Cue the ML to return to their seat(s).

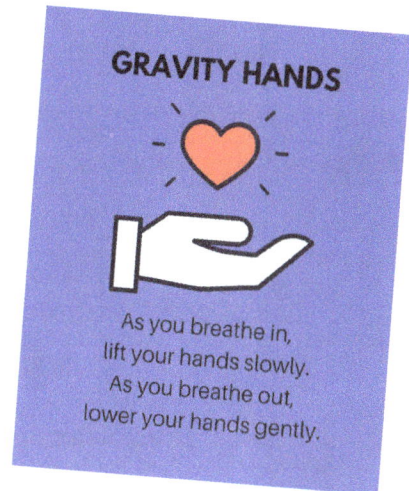

Going up and down the Conflict Escalator

Here are four options to help students explore what it feels like to go up and come down the Conflict Escalator using a series of conflict scenarios. Use the method or combination of methods that works best for your class.

1. Act it out: form student pairs (perhaps Peace Partners) to act out the Conflict Scenarios for the class.
2. Act it out: Teacher and a student act out Conflict Scenarios together
3. Read: form pairs (perhaps Peace Partners) and have students read the Conflict Scenarios from their seats.
4. Teacher reads out Conflict Scenarios

Draw an escalator on the board, copying the page in the resource section.

Have on hand two small magnets or post-it notes.

Decide how you want to engage in the Conflict Scenarios. Act out or read through each scenario two times.

The first time, just have the audience watch/listen.

The second time, ask the class to pretend they have a buzzer and to push the buzzer when they think the conflict is starting to go up the escalator.

Conflict scenario 1

Roles: Two siblings (1 and 2)

1: I'm hungry.

2: Me too. Let's see what's in the freezer.

1: Waffles!

2: Yes!

1: Oh no, there's only one left.

2: Are you sure there isn't another box?

1: Nope. Just this one waffle….

2: Are you going to eat it?

1: Yup.

2: That's not fair! You always get what you want!

1: No I don't! Don't be such a baby!

2: I'm not being a baby. You're being a pig.

1: You better give me that waffle!

2: Make me!

Note to teacher: The buzzer should go off when brother 2 says " You always get what you want!" Up until then the brothers are just calmly dealing with a conflict: there's only one waffle and two brothers want it.

Ask students to map the conflict on the escalator using a post-it note or a magnet to represent each brother.

You can draw the Conflict Escalator on the whiteboard or on some paper and have the kids fill in the steps (see example at end of lesson).

Conflict Scenario 2

Roles: two kids at school

Student 1: What do you want to do for our science project?

Student 2: We should do a test to see which paper towel is most absorbent.

Student 1: Oh I was thinking about doing something like do plants grow better when they are played classical music or hip hop.

Student 2: Huh. I guess that sounds okay but I really like the paper towel one.

Student 1: Yeah but my sister did that one and it wasn't that much fun.

Student 2: Well maybe your sister didn't do it right.

Student 1: Are you saying my sister is dumb?

Student 2: I don't know, is she?

Student 1: Not as dumb as you!

Note to teacher: The buzzer should go off when Student 1 says "Are you saying my sister is dumb?" Up until then the students are just calmly dealing with a conflict: they have two different ideas about what to do.

You can draw the Conflict Escalator on the whiteboard or on some paper and have the kids fill in the steps (see example).

Discuss

- What kinds of things cause a conflict to escalate? (tone of voice, insults, etc.)
- What part of your brain would be in charge when you start going up the conflict escalator? (amygdala)
- Would taking deep breaths help you to avoid escalating the conflict?

Say: *Over the next few lessons we'll learn a method to help work out conflicts if they have escalated.*

Peace Partners

Give students time to share what they did for the Peace Partners.

Do the Peace Partner activity as before.

Assign new Peace Partners. Remind your students that their job is to do at least one kind thing for their Peace Partner this week.

Closing words: *Okay, our time is up for today. Thank you for a great class, everyone.*

Optional: *Let's have a nice quiet moment for the bell. If you want to, you can close your eyes, picture your new Peace Partner, and imagine yourself doing something kind for them this week.*

The Conflict Escalator

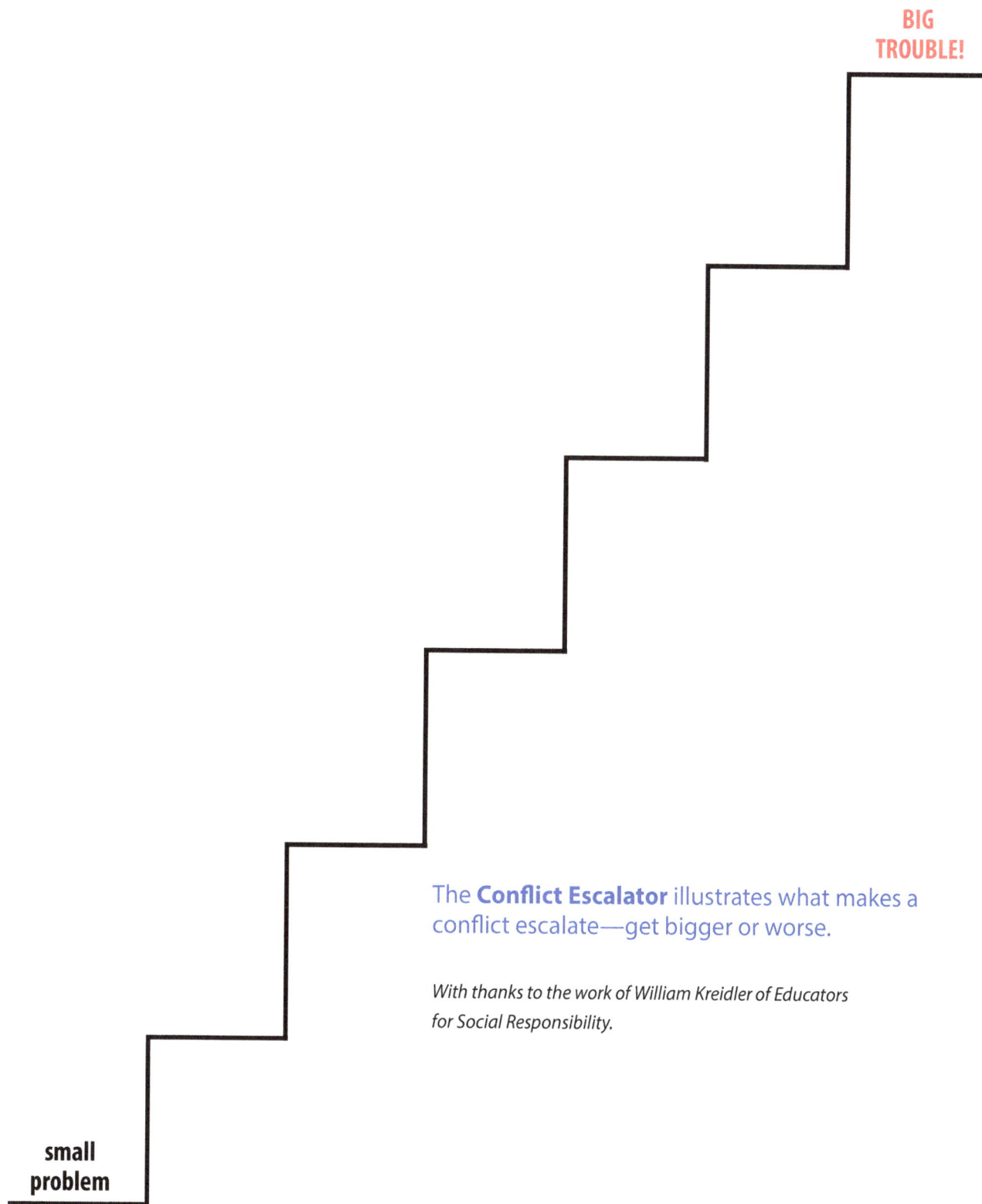

BIG TROUBLE!

The **Conflict Escalator** illustrates what makes a conflict escalate—get bigger or worse.

With thanks to the work of William Kreidler of Educators for Social Responsibility.

small problem

Lesson 16
MOFL or Awful?

OBJECTIVES: Explore methods to de-escalate conflicts

Explore what makes a good apology

Practice apologizing

Practice kindness

Assign new Peace Partners

PREPARATION: Review lesson

Your Peace Partners list

Copies of the MOFL worksheets found at the end of this lesson for each pair of students

Optional: bell or chime

Optional: student journals

Today we are going to be talking about a challenging and critical piece of effective conflict de-escalation: a good apology. We'll explore what makes a good apology using the shorthand MOFL: Mean it, Own It, Fix it, and Let it go. Before this lesson, you might reflect on your own relationship to apologizing and consider what you might share of your own experiences with your students. When did a good apology turn something around for you? When would it have helped?

Introduction

Say: *Last time we talked about what makes a conflict escalate. In order to work out a conflict, we have to take responsibility for whatever we did to make the conflict escalate. This can be hard because in general people don't like apologizing and most people are really bad at it. This lesson will help us to think more about how to apologize effectively.*

Mindfulness Practice

Invite today's Mindful Leader(s) (ML) to come to the front of the class.

Prompt the ML to say: "Let's sit up a little straighter. Close your eyes or look down into your lap. Let's take 3 deep breaths."

Say: Today I'm going to be describing some situations. Try to imagine that they are happening to you. Try to notice what you feel and if you can try to notice where you feel it in your body. Think back to when we did the lessons about where we feel emotions in our bodies. We're going to be trying that again.

Let's imagine…

You are bringing home an art project and someone bumps into you and knocks it out of your hands. It falls on the floor and breaks into pieces… How do you feel? Where in your body do you feel it?

You are bringing home an art project and someone bumps into you and knocks it out of your hands. The person turns around and says "Sorry!" and runs off. How do you feel? Where do you feel it?

You are bringing home an art project and someone bumps into you and knocks it out of your hands. The person turns around and sees what happened. They say "Oh my gosh I'm so sorry! I broke your project! Can I help you put it back together?" How do you feel? Where do you feel it?

Okay now let's think about this:

You borrowed a book from a friend and you accidentally spilled chocolate milk on some of the pages. How do you feel? Where do you feel it?

You wait for it to dry and you give it back to your friend and don't tell them about the milk. How do you feel? Where do you feel it?

You borrowed a book from a friend and you accidentally spilled chocolate milk on some of the pages. You give it back to your friend and say "Chocolate milk spilled on your book. Sorry!" How do you feel? Where do you feel it?

You borrowed a book from a friend and you accidentally spilled chocolate milk on some of the pages. You give them the book back and say "I spilled chocolate milk on your book. I'm really sorry! I will save up my money to get you a new one. I'm really sorry. How do you feel? Where do you feel it?

Pause.

After a few moments, say: *Now take one more deep breath in and out.*

Optional: Ask ML to ring the bell.

Ask students to open their eyes and/or look up when they are ready.

Cue the ML to return to their seat(s).

Discuss: Go over each scenario and ask kids to share how they were feeling.

MOFL: Mean it, Own it, Fix it, Leave it

Act out this scenario with a student in a few different ways:

Scenario 1: A student is drawing. You walk over and bump her so she messes up. She says, "Hey! You messed up my drawing!" You say, "Sorry!" and keep walking.

Ask: Is that a good apology? Why or why not?

Scenario 2. Act it out again but this time say "Sorry! I needed to get by" and keep walking.

Ask: Is that a good apology? Why or why not?

Scenario 3: Act it out again but this time say "Oh no! I'm so sorry! I wasn't watching where I was going. Can I help you fix it? I'm really sorry."

Ask: Is that a good apology? Why or why not?

Scenario 4: Act it out again, but this time say "Oh no! I'm so sorry! I wasn't watching where I was going. Can I help you fix it? I'm really sorry. Do you forgive me? You have to forgive me. I said I was sorry! Tell me that it's okay!"

Ask: Is that a good apology? Why or why not?

Write on the board: M O F L

Ask: Can anyone guess what the letters stand for? It has something to do with apologizing.

Explain that **the M stands for Mean it.** That a good apology has to be sincere and the person receiving it should see that you are truly sorry.

Ask: Why wasn't "Chocolate milk spilled on your book. Sorry." a good apology?

Somebody will probably say because the person didn't take responsibility for what they did. **The O in MOFL stands for Own it.** You have to take responsibility for what you did. Rather than saying "Mistakes were made" we would say. "I made a mistake."

Ask: When your art project was broken and the person apologized and offered to try to put it back together what were they doing? (trying to fix it)

> **The F stands for Fix it.** Even though it's not always possible, it's important to try to make amends and see if there is anything you can do to fix or remedy the situation.

Ask: Did it make the apology better when the person said "You have to forgive me!"?

> The **L stands for Let it Go**. Sometimes when people apologize they get very upset if the person receiving their apology doesn't accept it. It's important to remember that sometimes people aren't ready to forgive. Maybe they are still upset about what happened, even if they aren't really mad at you. We need to offer apologies and then let it go and let the person come to forgiveness when and if they are ready.

Ask the class to review the **four important parts of a good apology: Mean it, Own it, Fix it, Let it go.**

1. **Mean it** - show the person that you really regret what happened

2. **Own it** - in the meditation one apology was "Milk spilled on your book." Is that showing that you take responsibility for your actions? Do you have to take responsibility even if it was an accident? Give me an example

3. **Fix it** - what can you do to make things right?

4. **Let it go** - don't chase the person around making them forgive you. Sometimes that takes time - that isn't what this is about. This is about you offering something to the other person. You can't make them take it. But you do the right thing anyway. The only person you can control is yourself.

Apology Review with Peace Partners

Students will work with their Peace Partners to review some apologies.

- Students may act out the scenarios, or read through each apology, and then check off whether the apology shows that the person **means it, owns it, tries to fix it, and lets it go**.

- Ask them to circle the best apology.

- Have Peace Partners work together to complete both worksheets.

- After about five minutes, bring the group back together and have them share the pros and cons of each apology in terms of MOFL. Share what they think are the best apologies and why.

- You could ask: "MOFL or Awful?" :)

Peace Partners

Give students time to share what they did for the Peace Partners.

Do the Peace Partner activity as before.

Assign new Peace Partners. Remind your students that their job is to do at least one kind thing for their Peace Partner this week.

Closing words: *Okay, our time is up for today. Thank you for a great class, everyone.*

Optional: *Let's have a nice quiet moment for the bell. If you want to, you can close your eyes, picture your new Peace Partner, and imagine yourself doing something kind for them this week.*

MOFL Worksheet 1

1. Another student bumps into you when you are opening your locker and you drop your books. The student says: "Sorry! I was in a hurry to get in line."

   Mean it _____

   Own it _____

   Fix it _____

   Let it go _____

2. Another student bumps into you when you are opening your locker and you drop your books.

   The student says: "Sorry! You were in my way."

   Mean it _____

   Own it _____

   Fix it _____

   Let it go _____

3. Another student bumps into you when you are opening your locker and you drop your books.

   The student says: "Oh no! I'm sorry I knocked into you! Let me get your books for you!"

   Mean it _____

   Own it _____

   Fix it _____

   Let it go _____

4. Another student bumps into you when you are opening your locker and you drop your books.:

   The student says: "Oh no! I'm sorry! Let me help you pick up your books."

   You say: "That's okay. I'll just get them myself."

   The student says: "But I said I'm sorry! You have to accept my apology! Let me help you pick them up!!"

   Mean it _____

   Own it _____

   Fix it _____

   Let it go _____

Lesson 16
MOFL Worksheet 2

1. You are hurrying to line up for recess and you accidentally trip somebody and they fall down. They say, "Hey! You tripped me!" You say, "Sorry!"

   Mean it _____

   Own it _____

   Fix it _____

   Let it go _____

2. You are hurrying to line up for recess and you accidentally trip somebody and they fall down. They say, "Hey! You tripped me!" You say, "Oh sorry you fell. I was in a hurry."

   Mean it _____

   Own it _____

   Fix it _____

   Let it go _____

3. You are hurrying to line up for recess and you accidentally trip somebody and they fall down. They say, "Hey! You tripped me!" You say, "Oh I'm so sorry!! I was rushing and I wasn't watching where I was going. I'm really sorry. Are you okay? Do you want to get in front of me?"

   Mean it _____

   Own it _____

   Fix it _____

   Let it go _____

4. You are hurrying to line up for recess and you accidentally trip somebody and they fall down. They say, "Hey! You tripped me!" You say, ""Oh I'm so sorry!! I was rushing and I wasn't watching where I was going. I'm really sorry. Are you okay? Do you want to get in front of me?" They say, "No that's okay. Just leave me alone." You say, "Come on, I said I was sorry!!! Why are you still mad at me? It was just an accident. Geez."

   Mean it _____

   Own it _____

   Fix it _____

   Let it go _____

The Conflict CAT

OBJECTIVES:	Learn and practice using the Conflict CAT to resolve conflicts
	Engage students in mindfulness
	Practice kindness
	Assign new Peace Partners

PREPARATION:	Review lesson
	Your Peace Partners list
	6 Copies of the skit *Soccer vs. Basketball* found at end of lesson, if needed
	Optional: bell or chime
	Optional: student journals

This week we are going to learn a Conflict Resolution method called the Conflict CAT. CAT stands for Calm Down, Apologize, Toolbox. There is a diagram of the CAT at the end of the lesson. We have already learned how to use mindful breathing to **C**alm us down when our amygdalas take over. Last week we learned about how to **A**pologize effectively. Now we are going to focus on the **T**oolbox and learn about ways to work out conflicts.

Introduction

You might say: *Today we are going to put together many of the skills we've been practicing to de-escalate and solve conflicts. The method is called the Conflict CAT. The reason we learn about the CAT and practice it in class is so that you'll be ready when you need it in real life.*

One thing you'll notice is that it starts with mindfulness practice to help us calm down. In the real life moment when you need to calm down, you'll need to be able to do one of the mindfulness strategies we've been practicing. Today for our mindfulness practice, choose one of the practices that you feel works best for you. The more you practice, the easier it will be to use these tools in real life.

Mindfulness Practice

Invite today's Mindful Leader(s) (ML) to come to the front of the class.

Prompt the ML to say: "Let's sit up a little straighter. Close your eyes or look down into your lap. Let's take 3 deep breaths."

Invite students to choose their own practice: Take Five, Four Square, Gravity Hands, Clench and Release, Remote Control breathing or See Hear Feel.

After a few moments, say: *Now take one more deep breath in and out.*

Optional: Ask ML to ring the bell.

Ask students to open their eyes and/or look up when they are ready.

Cue the ML to return to their seat(s).

Putting the Conflict CAT to work

Here are three options to help students experience using the Conflict CAT.

1. Students act out the skit for the class.
2. Students read the skit aloud from their seats.
3. Students write their own skits, using this skit as a model.

Skit: Soccer vs. Basketball

Say: *We have a skit today called "Soccer vs. Basketball" that will help us experience what it's like to go up and down the conflict escalator.*

Ask for 6 volunteers to read or act out the skit. The characters are Dakota, Derrick, Dawson, Mateo, Zion, and Tamera. Hand them each a copy of the script.

Remind those not in the skit that they can notice where they are feeling emotions in their bodies as the skit unfolds.

You might also invite audience members to point a finger upward when the actors are going up the conflict escalator, and downward when they are making progress toward solving the conflict constructively.

Act/Read the skit.

Map the action of the skit conflict on the Conflict Escalator. Show how it went up and down.

Ask students to point out what made the conflict escalate and whether the apology was MOFL or Awful.

Ask what the kids did to finally work out the conflict. (They took turns.)

Ask them to brainstorm peaceful ways of working out this conflict. They could do something else like run around the track, Dawson could just be kind and play soccer, they could flip a coin, and so on.

Say: A quick way to help you remember how to work out a conflict peacefully is The Conflict C.A.T.

C stands for Calm Down
A stands for Apologize
T stands for Toolbox

Say: *We've already covered Calming Down (those are the mindfulness practices), we've talked about apologizing in Lesson 16 (MOFL or AWFUL). Today we're going to be focusing on the Toolbox.*

In the skit, what did the kids do to solve their problem in the end? (They took turns.)

Taking turns is one of the eight tools in the Conflict Toolbox. There are probably a million ways to work out a problem peacefully but today we're going to talk about 8 of them that you can try to remember to use in a conflict.

List and read over the 8 tools in the toolbox:

> **Taking Turns** - take turns using the object

> **Sharing** - share it

> **Being Kind** - let the other person have their way

> **Leave it to Chance** - flip a coin, rock, paper, scissors, etc.

Compromise - if you are arguing over what kind of pizza to have maybe you decide to eat pasta instead as long as you both like pasta

Pause the Conflict - if you are too angry to work things out take a while to calm down and then come back to working things out

Skip the Conflict - sometimes whatever you are having a conflict about isn't worth it going up the Conflict Escalator over. Or maybe you are trying to calm down and work things out but the other person keeps escalating. Sometimes you can just decide to walk away and skip the conflict because that is what is best for you.

Get Help - ask someone else to help you to work things out.

Conflict Scenarios

You might say: *I'm going to describe a conflict, and I want you to tell me which tool would work the best and why.*

Use the scenarios below or come up with your own situations that better reflect the needs of your class. Take a few answers for each one and discuss.

- You and a classmate both want to sit in the class comfy chair.
- You and your friend are arguing over what pizza topping to get.
- You and a friend can't agree on a movie to watch.
- You and a classmate are doing homework and you both need to use the classroom computer.

.Say: *Next time we are going to practice using the Conflict CAT to solve different problems. See if you find yourself in a conflict this week and see if you can use any of these tools.*

Peace Partners

Give students time to share what they did for the Peace Partners.

Do the Peace Partner activity as before.

Assign new Peace Partners. Remind your students that their job is to do at least one kind thing for their Peace Partner this week.

Closing words: *Okay, our time is up for today. Thank you for a great class, everyone.*

Optional: *Let's have a nice quiet moment for the bell. If you want to, you can close your eyes, picture your new Peace Partner, and imagine yourself doing something kind for them this week.*

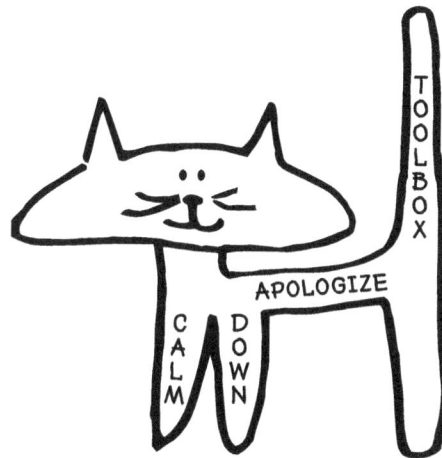

Lesson 17 SKIT
Soccer vs Basketball

Topic: Conflict Resolution
Characters: Dakota, Derrick, Dawson, Mateo, Tamera
Setting: at the park

_____

Dakota: Hey guys, let's play soccer!

Derrick: No, I want to play basketball.

Dawson: Me too. Soccer is for losers.

Zion: What?! Soccer is so cool!

Tamera: You're being mean, Dawson!

Dawson: No I'm not! Everybody knows that basketball is cooler than soccer!

Zion: Who cares about what's cooler? We're just here to have fun!

Dakota: All you care about is being cool, Dawson. You too, Derrick!

Derrick: I can't help it if you just like to do dorky things!

Dawson: Yeah, why don't you go play soccer with the other dorks?

Derrick: Good one, Dawson!

(**Derrick** and **Dawson** high five each other)

Mateo: Hey guys, we're going up the Conflict Escalator. Everybody is getting mad and our amygdalas are taking over.

Tamera: Mateo is right. We need to calm down.

Zion: Yeah that's right. Let's do that Take Five breathing we've been learning.

Derrick, Dawson, and Dakota: Well… okay.

They all do Take Five breathing

Mateo: Now that we're calm, maybe we can work out this conflict.

Derrick: Hey, Dakota, I'm sorry I made all those jokes about you being a dork.

Dawson: Yeah, me too. You're not a dork and soccer is fun. I just really felt like playing basketball.

Derrick: Yeah, me too. I'm sorry I got out of control.

Dakota: That's okay guys. We all flip our lids sometimes.

Zion: So what are we going to do?

Tamera: Maybe we should take turns. We could play soccer today and then play basketball tomorrow.

Mateo: Sounds good to me!

Derrick: Me too! Thanks guys.

Dakota: No problem! Let's go.

Derrick: I bet I make the most goals!

Dawson: No I can!

Mateo: Not again you guys…. No more conflicts!

Derrick and Dawson: Just kidding!

Everybody laughs.

The End

The Conflict Toolbox

1. SHARE
2. TAKE TURNS
3. BE KIND
4. LEAVE IT TO CHANCE

5. COMPROMISE
6. PAUSE THE CONFLICT
7. SKIP THE CONFLICT
8. GET HELP

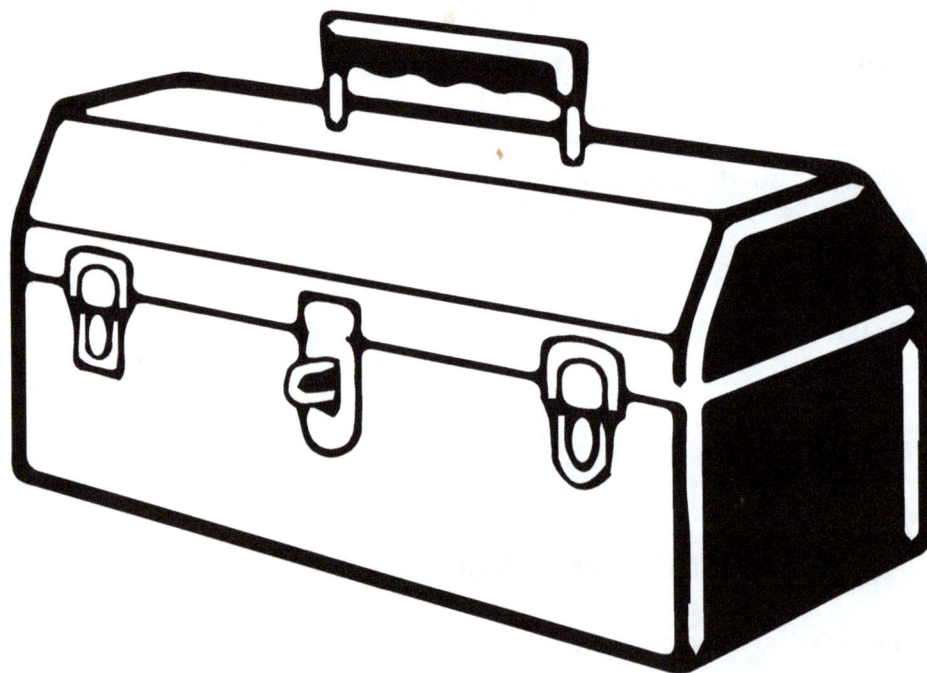

The Conflict CAT

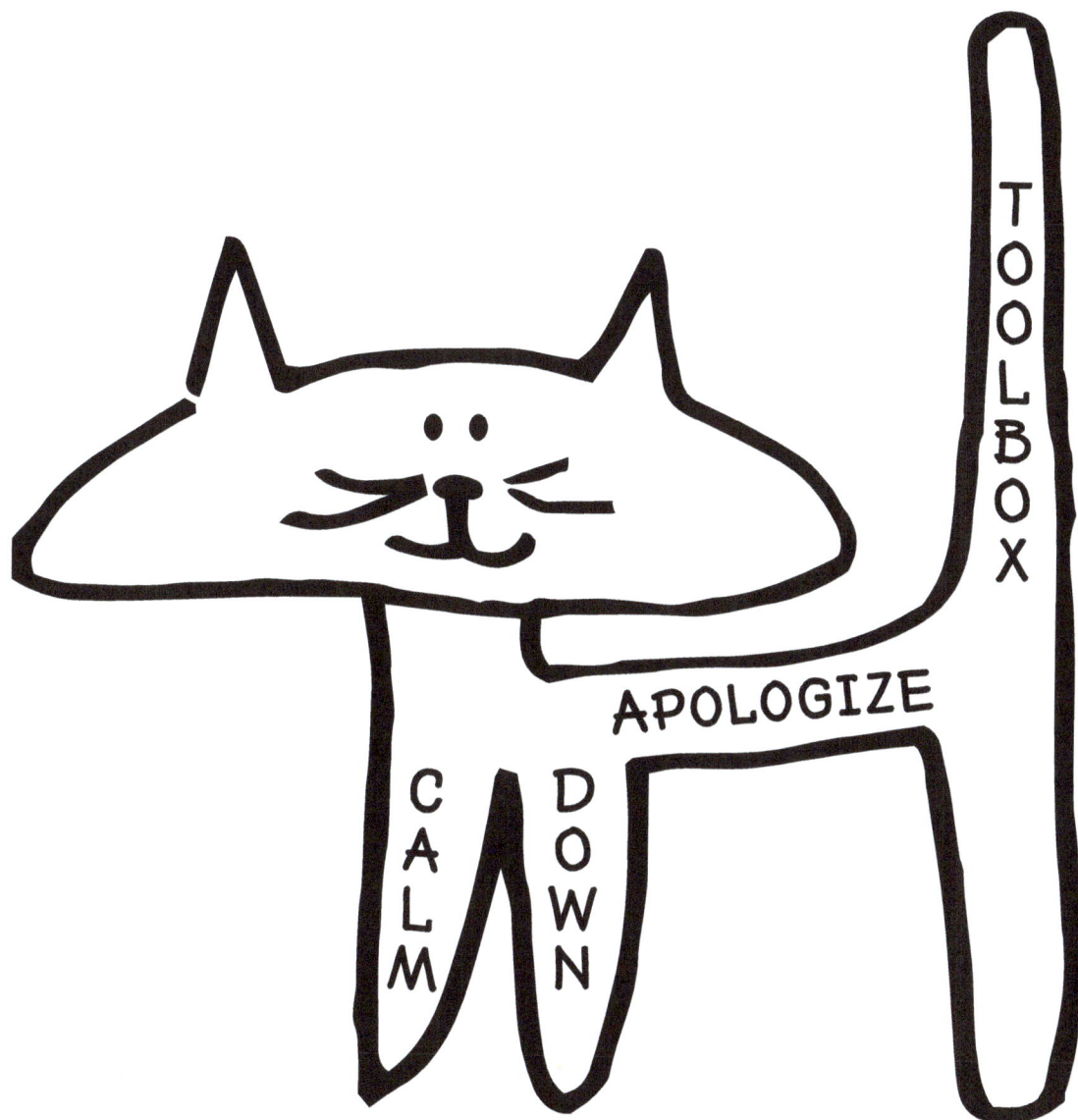

Lesson 18
Conflict Role Plays

OBJECTIVES: Practice using the Conflict CAT

Practice kindness

Assign new Peace Partners

PREPARATION: Review lesson

Your Peace Partners list

Slips of paper with one of the 4 conflict scenarios in the lesson written on each - enough for each pair of students to have one slip of paper.

Optional: Poster of the Conflict Escalator (page 115), Conflict CAT (page 131) and Toolbox (page 130) up where kids can see them.

Optional: bell or chime

Optional: student journals

Now that you have introduced and reviewed the three components of the Conflict CAT, the students are ready to put it to work. The more students practice using these tools when they are not really necessary - i.e., through skits and role plays - the more likely it is that they will be able to call on them when they are really needed.

Introduction

Say: *So we've learned a lot about working out conflicts so far. We've learned about how to use our breathing to help us to calm down. We've practiced apologizing in the skits that we've acted out. We've learned eight tools to use to work out conflicts. For today's challenge, let's see if we can put it all together.*

Mindfulness Practice

Invite today's Mindfulness Leader(s) (ML) to come to the front of the class.

Prompt the ML to say: "Let's sit up a little straighter. Close your eyes or look down into your lap. Let's take some deep breaths."

Invite students to choose their own practice: Take Five, Four Square, Gravity Hands, Clench and Release, Remote Control breathing or See Hear Feel.

After a few moments, say: *Now take one more deep breath in and out.*

Optional: Ask ML to ring the bell.

Ask students to open their eyes and/or look up when they are ready.

Cue the ML to return to their seat(s).

Practicing with the Conflict CAT

Review the Conflict CAT and the Toolbox Poster (or handouts).

Ask students to work with their Peace Partners.

You might say: *I am going to give each pair a conflict to work out in a role-play. You'll have a few minutes to work out how you are going to do it and to think about which tool you are going to use.*

Make sure that your role-play shows all the parts of the Conflict C.A.T.

1. Go up the Conflict Escalator BRIEFLY
2. One person says "We're going up the Conflict Escalator
3. One person says "Let's breathe" and do Take Five breathing
4. Both kids apologize for their role in escalating the conflict
5. Somebody offers a solution based on one of the tools.

Rules: no touching each other, no inappropriate language, teacher can use imaginary buzzer to cut off the escalation and get to the resolution.

Give each pair one of these conflict scenarios:

1. Two students disagree about who gets to be first in line
2. Two students disagree about who has the coolest shoes
3. Two students disagree about which NBA team is the best
4. There is only one slice of pizza left and two students want it.

Ring a bell to begin. Students begin to work out scenarios using the Conflict CAT.

Ring the bell again when time is up. Be flexible with the time.

> **NOTE:** *The real learning is coming from the practicing part of the process so don't rush it.*

Invite a few pairs to come up and show the class what they've come up with.

Make sure that they have covered all of the Conflict C.A.T. steps.

Written Reflection

Invite students to write a brief story inspired by a conflict scenario that includes all of the Conflict CAT elements: going up the escalator, calming down, apologizing, using a tool to solve the conflict. Students could also create a comic strip or story board.

Reflect and Discuss

1. What tools are you most likely to use?
2. What tools have you used before?
3. What parts of the CAT are easiest to use?
4. What parts of the CAT are hardest or most awkward to use?

Peace Partners

Give students time to share what they did for the Peace Partners.

Do the Peace Partner activity as before.

Assign new Peace Partners. Remind your students that their job is to do at least one kind thing for their Peace Partner this week.

Closing words: *Okay, our time is up for today. Thank you for a great class, everyone.*

Optional: *Let's have a nice quiet moment for the bell. If you want to, you can close your eyes, picture your new Peace Partner, and imagine yourself doing something kind for them this week.*

Lesson 19
Conflict CAT Game: Optional Lesson

OBJECTIVES: Practice Conflict Resolution skills

Engage students in mindfulness

Practice kindness

Assign new Peace Partners

PREPARATION: Review lesson

Your Peace Partners list

Posters of the Conflict Escalator (page 115), the
Conflict CAT (page 131) and the Conflict Toolbox
(page 130) up where kids can see them.

Conflict CAT Game sets for your whole class
(2-8 students per set)

Optional: bell or chime

Optional: student journals

If you feel that additional practice with the Conflict CAT would be useful, this
lesson can help. If you are ready to move on to Unit 6, you're welcome to do
that too.

Based on many years of work with students in the classroom, Peace of Mind
has developed a game that helps kids work together to put their mindfulness
practices, apologizing skills, and conflict resolution tools to work to solve
conflicts - and helps teachers see what their students have learned. Not surpris-
ingly, it's called the Conflict CAT Game.

PLEASE NOTE: The Conflict CAT game is really fun and kids enjoy playing it, but
buying it is optional. Each game is for 2-8 players. You would need enough sets
for your whole class to play at the same time. You might also just invest in one
set to have in your classroom for kids to play at other times. You can find out
more about the game at TeachPeaceofMind.org/shop/.

If you choose not to purchase the game, you can repeat Lesson 16 having the
kids work with a different partner with new scenarios.

Introduction

Say: *So we've learned a lot about working out conflicts so far. We've learned about how to use our breathing to help us to calm down. We've practiced apologizing in the skits that we've acted out. We've learned eight tools to use to work out conflicts.*

Today we're going to play a game that will help us see how skilled we have become at using what we've learned to solve conflicts.

The game is called- The Conflict CAT Game!

Mindfulness Practice

Invite today's Mindfulness Leader(s) (ML) to come to the front of the class.

Prompt the ML to say: "Let's sit up a little straighter. Close your eyes or look down into your lap. Let's take some deep breaths."

Invite students to choose their own practice: Take Five, Four Square, Gravity Hands, Clench and Release, Remote Control breathing or See Hear Feel.

After a few moments, say: *Now take one more deep breath in and out.*

Optional: Ask ML to ring the bell.

Ask students to open their eyes and/or look up when they are ready.

Cue the ML to return to their seat(s).

The Conflict CAT Game

You might say: *Today we are going to play a game that will help us to practice using the Conflict CAT method.*

Before we start the game we're going to talk about apologizing. In this game you are going to learn how to say "I'm sorry" in a bunch of different languages. Let's go over some of these together before we play.

Go over each card and have the kids repeat the words a few times.

Say: *Now let's get started. Here's how you play.*

Conflict CAT Game Directions:

Number of players per set: 2-8

Set up:

1. Separate cards into four piles: Conflicts, Mindfulness, Tools, Apologies
2. Place the cards face down on a table in four piles.
3. Decide who will be the first two actors.
4. Decide who will be the timer.

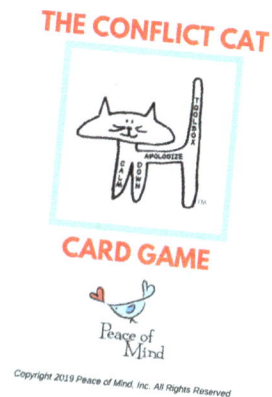

THE CONFLICT CAT

CARD GAME

Goal: Act out the conflict written on the card and solve the conflict using the mindfulness skill, tool, and apology on the cards you choose.

What you do:

1. The timer draws a card from each pile and turns them face up on the table.

2. The actors take a moment to look at the four cards that the timer has drawn.

3. The timer sets a timer (or just gets ready to count) to 10 seconds.

4. Timer says "Action!" and the actors start acting out the conflict - going up the Conflict Escalator.

5. After ten seconds the Timer says "Time!" and the actors have to start to work out the conflict.

6. One actor must say: "We're going up the Conflict Escalator!"

7. Then the actors role play working out the conflict by using the cards they have drawn: they do the mindfulness practice, they choose a language for an apology, and then they try to solve the conflict using one of the tools on the card.

> NOTE: *If neither of the tools is an appropriate way to solve the conflict then they can choose another "Tool" card.*

8. Once the conflict is resolved the players switch parts and play again.

If you have more kids you can spread out the jobs like Timer, Card-Drawer, Bell Ringer, etc.

It will be noisy with all of the groups playing at the same time. Walk around and see if it looks like they are following all of the steps. After each group has gone through all of the conflicts have them clean up the games and come back together as a group.

Reflect and Discuss

Prompt a discussion with these questions:

- How did that go?
- Did you have conflicts within your group while you were playing the Conflict CAT game?
- Were you able to work out those conflicts?
- Does anybody remember how to say "I'm Sorry" in a different language?
- Does anybody want to share how to say "I'm sorry" in a language that we didn't cover?

Say: *You now have skills that most people don't have. I hope that you will really try to start using these skills in your real life. Using these skills is pretty easy here in class but a lot more challenging when you are really angry.*

If everyone in our world knew how to work out conflicts like this, our world would be a much more peaceful place. I hope that you will use what you have learned so far in Peace Class to make your corner of the world more peaceful.

Peace Partners

Give students time to share what they did for the Peace Partners.

Do the Peace Partner activity as before.

Assign new Peace Partners. Remind your students that their job is to do at least one kind thing for their Peace Partner this week.

Closing words: *Okay, our time is up for today. Thank you for a great class, everyone.*

Optional: *Let's have a nice quiet moment for the bell. If you want to, you can close your eyes, picture your new Peace Partner, and imagine yourself doing something kind for them this week.*

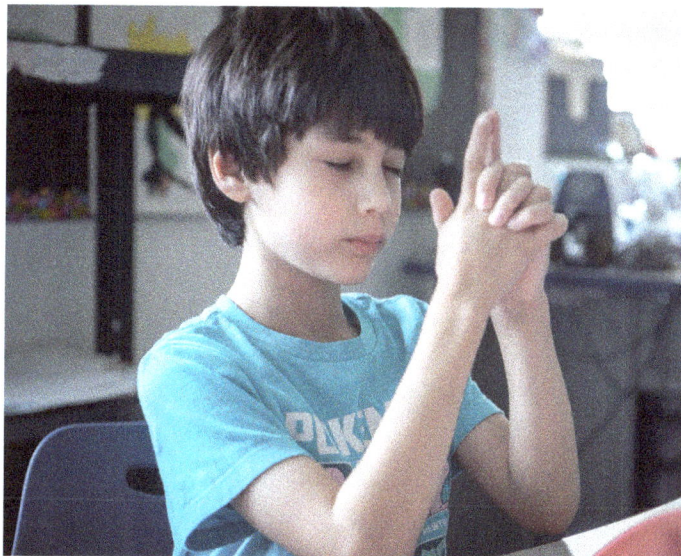

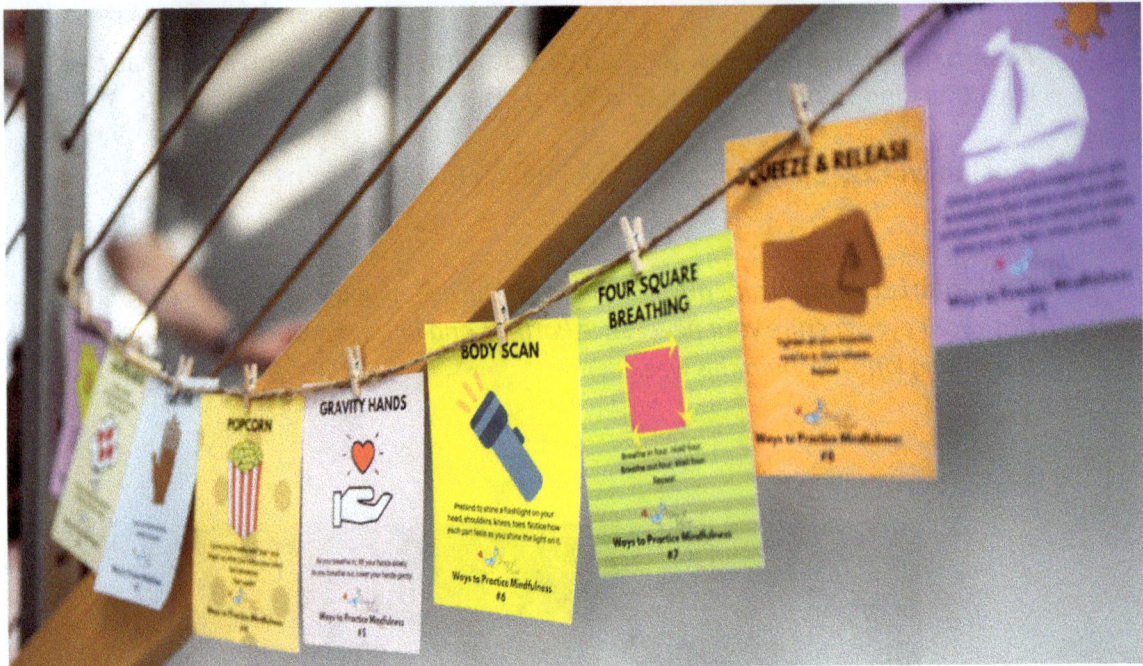

|

UNIT 6
Mindfulness for Social Justice

In this unit, we explore how mindfulness helps us to address stereotypes and implicit bias. We focus on the need for compassion for ourselves and others. We use mindfulness practices to develop metacognition skills to help us to become aware of our implicit bias. Students begin to explore how they can use what they've been learning to address societal challenges such as discrimination and racism.

Mindfulness for Social Justice

When you talk about stereotypes and bias, racism and sexism with your students, it will be helpful to frame the conversation in the context of broader societal forces of power and oppression. You might point out that if a group of people has more power in our society, then stereotypes the powerful group may believe about the group that has less power may be used to harm them, either on purpose or without realizing it.

As Ijeoma Oluo says, "Racism is any prejudice against someone because of their race, when those views are reinforced by systems of power."[1]

To talk constructively about sexism, it helps to understand the historical and structural power differences between men and women. To have a constructive conversation about race, it helps to understand how our society's history of structural racial inequality impacts our lives today.

The good news is, mindfulness practice, combined with an understanding of our brains, kindness and gratitude practice, empathy and compassion, equips us to do this work in transformative ways - for ourselves and for our communities.

In this unit, we have drawn on the work and wisdom of Dena Simmons, Zaretta Hammond, Dr. Ibram X. Kendi, Robin DiAngelo, Ijeoma Oluo, Tovi Scruggs-Hussein and Rhonda Magee among many others. Please see the Resources section to find links to their work.

---

1   Oluo, Ijeoma, *So you want to talk about race* (Seal Press, 2019) 26.

Unit 6 Terms

In the lessons that follow, we use these terms with these meanings. This glossary is to help you prepare to teach, not necessarily to share with your students.

Anti-racism: taking action to dismantle racist systems.

Bias: prejudice in favor of or against one thing, person, or group compared with another, usually in a way considered to be unfair.

Discrimination: action based on prejudice including ignoring, threatening, excluding or being violent toward another person or group of people.

Gender: socially constructed characteristics of masculinity and femininity, such as norms, roles, and relationships of and between groups of women and men. It varies from society to society and can be changed.

Gender expression: how we express our gender identity through clothing, hairstyles, accessories.

Gender Identity: a deeply held sense of being male, female or another gender or no gender. Gender identity is not related to sexual orientation.

Implicit Bias: the attitudes or stereotypes that affect our understanding, actions, and decisions in an unconscious manner.

Intersectionality: each of us has multiple identities, including gender, class, sexuality, and race, and there are privileges and oppressions that come with each of these aspects of our experiences. It is important to keep the interactions of those in mind.

Microaggressions: according to author Ijeoma Oluo, microaggressions are "small daily insults and indignities perpetrated against marginalized or oppressed people because of their affiliation with that marginalized or oppressed group."

Non-Binary: applies to people who do not feel like the words "girl" or "boy" fit. They may feel like both or neither. They sometimes use pronouns such as they, them, theirs.

Prejudice: pre-judgment about another person based on the groups to which that person belongs. This includes stereotypes, attitudes and generalizations that are based on little or no experience.

Privilege: according to author Ijeoma Oluo: "Privilege, in the social justice context, is an advantage or a set of advantages that you have that others do not." This advantage might come from your race, economic class, sexuality, physical abilities, and so on. So "white privilege" would refer to the advantages a white person has living in a society that favors and normalizes whiteness, which can keep them from seeing and understanding the disadvantages and struggles of people of color in the same society.

Race: a social construct, an evolving social idea that was created to legitimize racial inequality and protect white advantage.

Racism: a system in which one racial group's prejudice is backed by legal authority and institutional control.

Racialized Identity: the way in which people are seen based on what race they are perceived to be.

Sex: refers to biological reproductive organs and sex chromosomes.

Sexism: a system in which one gender's prejudice is backed by legal authority and institutional control.

Sexual Orientation: an inherent or immutable enduring emotional, romantic or sexual attraction to other people.

Stereotypes: widely held cultural beliefs, images and distorted truths about a group of people.

Systemic Racism: a political or social system based on racism.

Transgender or Trans: applies when your gender identity (how you feel) is different than what doctors/midwives assigned to you when you were born (girl/boy or sex assigned at birth).

Definitions drawn from these sources:

Ijeoma Oluo: *So You Want to Talk About Race*
Robin DiAngelo *White Fragility*
Teaching Tolerance
World Health Organization

Lesson 20
Compassion for ourselves and others

OBJECTIVES: Learn a new mindfulness practice called Heartfulness

Practice compassion for ourselves and others

Engage students in mindfulness

Practice kindness

Assign new Peace Partners

PREPARATION: Review lesson

Your Peace Partners list

Prepare to show the video: Unsung Hero https://www.youtube.com/watch?v=uaWA2GbcnJU[2]

Optional: bell or chime

Optional: student journals

In this lesson, we will learn a new mindfulness practice called Heartfulness and practice compassion toward ourselves and others. As Oren Sofer, author of *Say What You Mean: A Mindful Approach to Nonviolent Communication*, says:

> *Loving-kindness (or heartfulness) practice transforms bias in a different way. The cultivation of prosocial mental states like kindness and compassion alters the default internal atmosphere of the heart/mind towards an innate disposition of goodwill. This may have the effect of overriding or replacing implicit bias. Initial studies have shown that six weeks of loving-kindness, even seven minutes of this intentional practice, can reduce implicit bias.*

This is an important foundational practice for the lessons to come, especially for lessons on addressing implicit bias. Use this practice as needed throughout the rest of the curriculum.

---

2   Today we have included a video on compassion made by a Thai Insurance Company. We are in no way endorsing the company or their products, nor do we have any relationship with the company of any kind.

Background reading: Why is it so important to address implicit bias in our teaching? Educator and author Zaretta Hammond explains why it's important, what works, and what doesn't. Four Tools for Interrupting Implicit Bias

Introduction

Say: *In this next unit we are going to be doing some challenging work. We'll be talking about some of the most difficult problems facing our society - sexism, racism, implicit bias, stereotypes and unkind actions stemming from these problems. We'll be exploring all of those things over the next several lessons. To get us more ready to take on these challenges together, we're going to learn a compassion practice. Compassion practices have been shown to increase empathy and decrease bias.*

When we do compassion practices, we try to think about ourselves and other people and we think some kind thoughts for them. We're not saying these things out loud or even telling people that we were thinking of them. This is just something that we are trying out in our own minds. We're just trying to see what it feels like and to see if over time it changes the way we feel about other people and ourselves.

Sometimes it can be hard to think kind thoughts about ourselves. Have you ever noticed that? If I asked you right now to say, "I'm awesome!" How would you feel?

Take some answers from the class.

What if I asked you to say "I deserve to be happy?" What would that feel like?

Take some answers from the class.

Some of you might feel uncomfortable or even selfish thinking kind thoughts about yourself. That's fine. Any way that you feel is fine. But just try this as an experiment.

Research shows that people who are kind to themselves are much more likely to be kind to other people. So maybe you can think about being kind to yourself as something you are doing for other people.

Okay - let's try it. As always this is optional. If you want to sit quietly and think about something else that is always your choice.

MIndfulness Practice

Invite today's Mindfulness Leader(s) (ML) to come to the front of the class.

Prompt the ML to choose another student to turn off the classroom lights.

Prompt the ML to say: "Let's sit up a little straighter. Let's close our eyes/ or leave them open, looking at the floor in front of you. Let's take 3 deep breaths."

Heartfulness for someone who makes you happy

I'd like you to think about someone who makes you happy. Someone you see every day, at home or at school, could be someone in your family, a friend, a teacher, even a pet. Just choose someone and try to picture them happy and smiling. Picture them doing something that makes them happy. Try to notice how you feel when you think about this person.

Now, if you'd like to, put your hand over your heart and repeat these words in your mind while you think about this person:

May you be happy. **Pause.**

May you be healthy. **Pause.**

May you be peaceful. **Pause**.

Take a moment to notice how you feel. Any way that you feel is fine, even if you feel nothing. Just try to notice it.

Heartfulness for yourself

Say: *This might feel a little strange, but this time we are going to send kind thoughts to ourselves. Imagine yourself happy and smiling, doing something that you like to do. Now repeat these words in your mind.*

May I be happy. **Pause**.

May I be healthy. **Pause**.

May I be peaceful. **Pause.**

Again, try to notice how you feel. Does it feel different to send kind thoughts to yourself? Any way that you feel is fine. Just try to notice it.

Heartfulness for someone who you are a little bit mad at

Say: *Now I'd like you to think about someone you are mad at, or someone who made you feel sad. See if you can choose someone that you are just a little bit mad at. Maybe your brother ate the last bowl of cereal or your sister lost your page in the book you were reading. Not somebody who makes you really angry.*

Once you have chosen someone try to picture them happy and smiling. Picture them doing something that makes them happy. Try to notice how you feel when you think about this person. Remember, they can't hear you. You are just trying to notice how it feels to think these thoughts or feel these feelings. This is for you.

Now, if you'd like to, put your hand over your heart and repeat these words in your mind while you think about this person:

May you be happy. **Pause.**

May you be healthy. **Pause.**

May you be peaceful. **Pause**.

Take a moment to notice how you feel. Any way that you feel is fine, even if you feel nothing. Just try to notice it.

Heartfulness for each other

Finally we are just going to be thinking about each other and about everyone in the world. Just try to notice what image comes up in your mind when you think about "everyone in the world."

Now, if you'd like to, put your hand over your heart and repeat these words in your mind while you think about this person:

May we all be happy. **Pause.**

May we all be healthy. **Pause.**

May we all be peaceful. **Pause.**

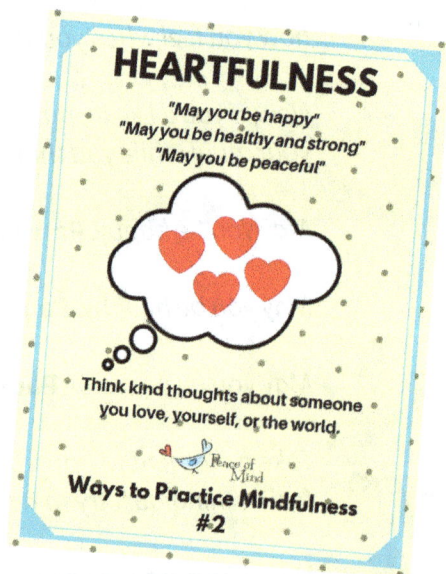

HEARTFULNESS

"May you be happy"
"May you be healthy and strong"
"May you be peaceful"

Think kind thoughts about someone you love, yourself, or the world.

Peace of Mind

Ways to Practice Mindfulness #2

After a few moments, say: *Now take one more deep breath in and out.*

Optional: Ask ML to ring the bell.

Ask students to open their eyes and/or look up when they are ready.

Cue the ML to return to their seat(s).

Reflect and Discuss

- What was that like for you?
- Does anybody want to share who you were thinking about?
- What did it feel like to think kind thoughts about yourself?
- What did it feel like to think kind thoughts about someone you are annoyed with?

Heartfulness and Kindness Practice

The following are some activities that can go along with the Heartfulness practice. Research shows that compassion practices like these help us to practice kindness towards ourselves and others.

You can choose to do some or all of these activities within this lesson or any time you want to inspire kindness and build community.

1. Unsung Hero Video

This is a life insurance commercial from Thailand that has a beautiful message about the power of small kindnesses. A man is seen doing little acts of kindness in his community and getting no credit for them. He is even seen as weak and silly by some of the people who observe him. To set the tone for the following activities, or just to experience a reminder of the power of small acts of kindness, this video can be inspirational. "Unsung Hero" https://www.youtube.com/watch?v=uaWA2GbcnJU

Discuss

1. Name some of the acts of kindness shown in this video.
2. Why did the man do these kind things?
3. What did he get out of doing these kind things?

4. Why did the other shopkeepers shake their heads at him?

5. What happened to the little girl who was asking for money for school?

You might explain that in our country we have free public schools but that in some other countries there are only private schools and so many children do not get a chance to go to school if they cannot afford it.

2. Kindness Chain

Directions for the Class:

1. Sit in a circle or as close to that as possible.

2. Think of something kind to say about the person on your right.

3. Take a moment to think about that person.

4. We are not going to be talking about people's appearance so we won't be saying things like "I like your hair" or "your sweatshirt is cool."

5. Instead, try to think about something that you know and admire about this person. Some examples could be "You make people laugh," "You always seem to try really hard," "I've noticed that you are a good friend to people," "You are very helpful," "You are great at drawing (or music, or math, or sports, etc.)."

> **NOTE:** *Some kids will feel uncomfortable with this activity so make sure to give students the opportunity to pass.*

You might say: *Sometimes, even if I'm sitting next to my best friend, my mind might go blank and I can't think of anything to say. If that happens to you just say that you need help and I'll choose someone else or I'll say something kind about that person myself. But we're all going to really try to do this.*

If students pass, you can ask for a volunteer to say something kind about this student.

After you go around the circle go back around the other way.

3. Alternative Kindness Chain Activity

If you think your students might not be comfortable saying these things in person, another way to do this is to have each student have a large index card taped to their back. Students can take turns going around and writing something kind on each person's card anonymously. Make sure to set expectations about kindness and give warnings about how joke comments can sometimes be misconstrued. Encourage earnest comments.

Discuss

- What did it feel like to say something kind about someone else?
- What did it feel like to have someone say something kind about you?
- If you did the face-to-face version of the activity: Did it feel uncomfortable in any way to give or receive these compliments? Why do you think that is?
- If you did the index card activity: What did it feel like to be able to give compliments anonymously? Did you feel more free to express yourself? Do you wish that you could tell the other person which compliment was from you?
- What else did you notice or want to share?

Peace Partners

Give students time to share what they did for the Peace Partners.

Assign new Peace Partners. Remind your students that their job is to do at least one kind thing for their Peace Partner this week.

Closing words: *Okay, our time is up for today. Thank you for a great class, everyone.*

Optional: *Let's have a nice quiet moment for the bell. If you want to, you can close your eyes, picture your new Peace Partner, and imagine yourself doing something kind for them this week.*

Lesson 21
Fast and Slow Thinking

OBJECTIVES:
Learn about "Fast and Slow Thinking" and relate concept to earlier lessons

Explore the pros and cons of fast and slow thinking

Engage students in mindfulness

Practice kindness

Assign new Peace Partners

PREPARATION:
Review lesson

Your Peace Partners list

6 copies of the skit *The Story I'm Telling Myself* found at the end of the lesson, if needed

Prepare to show the video, being careful to choose your starting point to skip YouTube ads: <u>Brain Tricks - This Is How Your Brain Works.</u> Written and created by Mitchell Moffit and Gregory Brown of ASAP Science. https://www.youtube.com/watch?v=JiTz2i4VHFw

Optional: bell or chime

Optional: student journals

In this lesson, we introduce the concept of Fast and Slow Thinking that Nobel Laureate Daniel Kahneman explores in his book *Thinking, Fast and Slow*. This approach gives students another way to understand the role of the amygdala and the PFC and to review what they've learned about the brain's negativity bias. It also emphasizes the value of the mindfulness practice of noticing our thoughts (see Remote Control Breathing in Lesson 8), and taking time to consider whether what we are thinking is really true.

Introduction

You might say: *One benefit of learning to notice and pay attention to our thoughts is that this practice gives us an opportunity to notice what the story is that we're telling ourselves about a situation, and to ask if the story is really true. Is what I'm assuming really true? Is it false? Or do I just not know?*

Today we are going to learn about the ways our brain thinks fast and thinks slow. It's really amazing how our brain works - we'll get a little more insight. When it comes to how we treat other people, sometimes our fast thinking can get us into trouble - we'll explore that too.

But first, our mindfulness practice. As always this is optional. If you want to sit quietly and think about something else that is always your choice.

Mindfulness Practice

Invite today's Mindfulness Leader(s) (ML) to come to the front of the class.

Prompt the ML to say: "Let's sit up a little straighter. Close your eyes or look down into your lap. Let's take 3 deep breaths."

Repeat *the Remote Control Breathing practice from Lesson 8.*

After a few moments, say: *Now take one more deep breath in and out.*

Optional: Ask ML to ring the bell.

Ask students to open their eyes and/or look up when they are ready.

Cue the ML to return to their seat(s).

Fast and Slow Thinking

Say: *Today we are going to be learning something new about our brains. Researchers have discovered that our brains have two ways of thinking - fast and slow - also known as System 1 (fast) and System 2 (slow).*

Our fast brain (System 1) is our "gut reaction" when we react without thinking. Does this sound familiar? We learned about a part of our brain that operates without thinking -- the amygdala. The amygdala is like our threat detection center and is incredibly important for keeping us safe.

Our slow brain (system 2) is the way of thinking that reflects on things, takes in the information, and makes decisions. This sounds a bit like what the PFC does.

Ask: Can you think of an example of fast thinking that would be helpful?

Offer an example: *You see a ball coming toward you and you cover your face or quickly try to catch it.*

Ask: Would slow thinking be helpful in that scenario?

Answer: *No, you don't want to think too hard about a ball that is coming at you. You want to react quickly.*

Ask: *Can you think of an example of fast thinking that would be unhelpful?*

Take some answers and offer an example:

- Maybe there is a new kid in your class and he is wearing a Yankees baseball jersey. You are a Boston Red Sox fan and those two teams have a longstanding rivalry.
- What might your fast thinking brain decide about that kid?

  That he loves the Yankees, therefore he hates the Red Sox, therefore he is not on your side, therefore you don't want to be friends with him.

- What would your slow thinking decide?

  Hey that kid is wearing a Yankees jersey. I wonder if he likes baseball as much as I do? Maybe I'll go ask him if he likes to play baseball…

- Then maybe when you ask him, he says that it is his brother's jersey and he doesn't really like the Yankees - that he's more into soccer.

Say: *That is an example of how we might get things totally wrong about people and situations when we go only by fast thinking.*

We're lucky that our brains have the capacity to do fast and slow thinking. When it comes to how we treat other people, sometimes our fast thinking, System 1 thinking can become a problem.

Do you remember when we learned about the Negativity Bias? How it can be really helpful in keeping us safe but can also cause us to forget about and not notice so many good things in our lives? Fast thinking can also cause us sometimes to make snap judgements about people that can be wrong and harmful.

Watch Video

Say: *Let's watch a video that will help us understand Fast and Slow thinking. I'll be stopping the video every once in a while so that we can do the activities.*

Watch the video: <u>Brain Tricks - This Is How Your Brain Works</u> https://www.youtube.com/watch?v=JiTz2i4VHFw

Stop the video at **00:39** and have the class guess which line is the longest.

Resume the video.

Stop the video at **1:08** when it gets to the brain test and have the students try it in real time. They will need a pencil and paper or their journals.

Resume the video.

Stop the video at **2:11** when it gets to the bat and ball test and have them try to answer the question.

Resume the video

Stop the video at **2:45** after the question about Moses and the Ark - take some answers.

Resume the video.

Discuss: Fast thinking makes you think "What you see is all there is" - WYSIATA.[3]

- Can you think of examples of WYSIATA?
- Write or share about a time when your first reaction to something (like a food or an activity) or to a person turned out to be wrong. Write or share your thoughts with a partner.

The Story I'm Telling Myself

Choose from one of the following approaches:

1. Students act out the The Story I'm Telling Myself skit
2. Students read tThe Story I'm Telling Myself skit aloud from their seats
3. Teacher reads the skit aloud and class discusses

---

3   Kahneman, D. *Thinking, Fast and Slow* (New York: Farrar, Straus and Giroux, 2015)

Introduce the skit: *Today we are going to be [acting out/ reading/ listening to] a skit about how fast thinking can lead us to make up stories that aren't really true. This is something that almost everybody does, but once we start to notice it we can try to decide if the story we're telling ourselves is helpful to us or not.*

For options 1 and 2, choose 6 actors to play Julio, Hassan, Tianna, Mom, Narrator 1 and Narrator 2. **Hand out** copies of the skit and have them act it out or read it.

Instruct the audience to notice examples of fast and slow thinking in the skit.

Act/Read/Listen to the skit.

Reflect and Discuss

- Was Hassan doing fast or slow thinking when he heard his friends talking about his song?
- Why didn't he challenge his fast thinking when he was talking to his mom about it?
- What would you have done if you thought that you heard your friends saying something mean about you?
- Can you think of a time when you believed something about someone that didn't turn out to be true?
- How could mindfulness help you to take a moment to do some slow thinking?

DON'T BELIEVE EVERYTHING YOU THINK!

Peace Partners

Give students time to share what they did for the Peace Partners.

Assign new Peace Partners. Remind your students that their job is to do at least one kind thing for their Peace Partner this week.

Closing words: *Okay, our time is up for today. Thank you for a great class, everyone.*

Optional: *Let's have a nice quiet moment for the bell. If you want to, you can close your eyes, picture your new Peace Partner, and imagine yourself doing something kind for them this week.*

Lesson 21
Skit: The Story I'm Telling Myself

Topic: Fast and slow Thinking
Characters: Julio, Hassan, Tianna, Mom, Narrator 1, Narrator 2
Setting: Outside Tianna's front door and Hassan's house

_____

Narrator 1: Hassan, Tianna and Julio are really good friends. They like to play music together and write their own songs.

Narrator 2: One day Hassan went over to Tianna's house and was about to knock on the door when he heard Hassan and Tianna talking.

Narrator 1: He couldn't hear them very well through the door but he listened for a minute. This is what he thought he heard.

Tianna: I think Hassan's new song is really bad.

Julio: Yeah me too.

Hassan: *(Feeling really hurt and mad)* Man that's so mean!

Narrator 2: Hassan turned around and ran home.

Later at Hassan's house

Hassan's Mom: Hassan what's wrong? You look really upset.

Hassan: Nothing. I'm just mad because of something that happened this afternoon.

Mom: What happened?

Hassan: Well, I heard Tianna tell Julio that my new song really is really bad.

Mom: Really? That doesn't sound like Tianna….

Hassan: Well it is. She's really mean. I don't think I want to be friends with her anymore.

Mom: Wow that's pretty extreme. Don't you think you should talk to her about it?

Hassan: No. She obviously doesn't like any of my songs and has been lying to me this whole time. She's a liar. And Julio said he "totally agrees." What a jerk.

Mom: Really? You've known Tianna and Julio for a long time. They always seem like really good friends.

Hassan: Well, they're not.

Mom: Huh. Well I still think you should talk to them. (walks away)

Narrator 2: The next day:

Narrator 1: Julio and Tianna come over to Hassan's house to pick him up to go to school.

Julio: Hey Hassan!

Hassan:

Tianna: Good morning Hassan!

Hassan: **Tianna**: Hassan, I said Good morning. What's up?

Hassan: Nothing.

Julio: Okay…. hey, Tianna and I are thinking we should try out for the school talent show.

Tianna: Yeah.

Hassan: Uh, no thanks. I'm not interested.

Tianna: What? We've been talking about this for weeks…

Julio: Yeah - we can do my new song.

Tianna: No, we should do Hassan's new song.

Hassan: What? **My** new song?!

Tianna: Yeah - it's really good!

Hassan: You're lying! Yesterday I heard you tell Julio that you thought it was really bad!

Tianna: What?! I did not! I said that your new song was really "rad"! It's great!

Hassan: Wait, I'm really confused. I totally thought you said it was bad.

Tianna: Why would I say that? That's really mean.

Julio: Geez Hassan - we wouldn't say that.

Hassan: Wow. I had that totally wrong. I just reacted to what I thought I heard and didn't stop to think about it at all. I'm really sorry you guys.

Tianna: No problem!

Julio: Let's go practice your new song!

Hassan: Awesome!

The End

Lesson 22
Like a What?

OBJECTIVES:

Explore stereotypes and bias

Engage students in mindfulness

Establish terms

Practice kindness

Assign new Peace Partners

PREPARATION:

Review lesson

Your Peace Partners list

Prepare to show the video, being careful to choose your starting point to skip YouTube ads: *Run Like a Girl* https://youtu.be/XjJQBjWYDTs[4]

Optional: bell or chime

Optional: student journals

Books, computer games, the Web, television - there are so many places that we can be exposed to stereotypes, that we can be exposed to distorted information. And there is a whole universe of information that we're not getting. Think about these stereotypes, these omissions, these distortions as a kind of environment that surrounds us, like smog in the air. We don't breathe it because we like it. We don't breathe it because we think it's good for us. We breathe it because it's the only air that's available.

— Dr. Beverly Daniel Tatum
Author of Why Are All the Black Kids Sitting Together
in the Cafeteria?: And Other Conversations About Race

This lesson addresses stereotypes, focusing specifically on stereotypes about girls. The video called "Run like a Girl" offers a helpful introduction to the topic. You might like to watch this before class and notice where the timing cues are. We will explore how mindfulness can help us approach these topics with

---

4   "Run Like a Girl" is made by a company that sells products to girls and women. We are in no way endorsing the product or the company, nor do we have any relationship with the company of any kind.

compassion for ourselves and others. Mindfulness helps to notice that thoughts and biases are just thoughts, not facts. If we can notice that we have them, then we can take some time to decide if we actually believe them or not.

We are also going to present a list of terms that will be used in the following lessons.

Recommended Reading: To help prepare for this lesson, take a few minutes to review these helpful resources from Teaching Tolerance and The Trevor Project. https://www.thetrevorproject.org/https://www.tolerance.org/magazine/summer-2013/the-gender-spectrum

Introduction

You might say: *Today we are going to be noticing our thoughts and learning about how our thoughts can affect the way we think about and treat others. We'll be thinking about fast and slow thinking and applying what we've learned to discussing gender stereotypes.*

But let's start with our mindfulness practice. Are you starting to see that learning how to notice your thoughts and to pause and pay attention to what you are thinking can be helpful?

Mindfulness Practice

Invite today's Mindfulness Leader(s) (ML) to come to the front of the class.

Prompt the ML to say: "Let's sit up a little straighter. Close your eyes or look down into your lap. Let's take 3 deep breaths."

Repeat Remote Control Breathing practice from Lesson 8.

After a few moments, say: *Now take one more deep breath in and out.*

Optional: Ask ML to ring the bell.

Ask students to open their eyes and/or look up when they are ready.

Cue the ML to return to their seat(s).

Discuss

Take a moment to let students share what they were noticing in their minds today.

Ask:

- Did your mind's remote control change the channel?
- What did you end up "watching?"
- Were you able to change the channel back to the "Breathing Channel?"

Reflecting on Stereotypes

Say: *Today we are going to be talking about stereotypes. When I say, "All girls like the color pink." What do you think? Is this true?*

Take some answers.

Most of you think that this is not true. While it is true that some people like the color pink, including some girls, it is not true that **all** *girls like the color pink. But if you were to go to a store and look at the toy or clothing sections - especially for little kids - what color would you see the most in the "girls" section?*

Take some answers.

That's right, pink. Somehow, over the course of time pink has become associated with girls and there is an assumption that girls like pink things. So when I say, "All girls like pink" that is a widely held belief about a group of people that may be true for some of them but is definitely not true for all of them. That is what we call a stereotype.

While "all girls like pink" isn't a very harmful stereotype, many stereotypes are very harmful and can lead to discrimination and cruelty. Over the next two lessons we're going to be talking about stereotypes that have to do with gender.

Let's talk about gender

Say: *Before we get started let's go over some terms. These terms can be confusing and people don't all agree on them. But these are the definitions that we are going to use here.*

 | https://TeachPeaceofMind.org

When we say **gender** we are talking about whether someone is male, female, **non-binary** or **gender fluid**. You might not be familiar with those two last terms. While most people are most familiar with gender as being male or female, gender is actually more of a **spectrum**. Although the concept of a gender spectrum and the fact that some people don't identify as male or female may be unfamiliar ideas, they aren't new. There are lots of examples of non-binary or gender fluid people in history, and today more and more people are publicly identifying as being on the gender spectrum.

A person's **gender identity** is a deeply held sense of being male, female, another gender or no gender.

Gender identity is not related to **sexual orientation.** Sexual orientation is about who someone is attracted to or loves.

Sometimes when a person's gender identity (how they feel) doesn't match the gender that they were assigned by their doctor when they were born, they are **transgender.**

Gender expression is how we express our gender identity through our clothing, hairstyle, or accessories.

Students' experience with stereotypes

Say: So, gender stereotypes are ideas that people have about how people will, or sometimes how people should, act based on their gender.

Ask: Can you think of examples of gender stereotypes that you have heard?

For example:

- All girls like princesses
- All women love babies
- Boys don't cry
- Men like football

Take some more examples and discuss. You might point out that while these things are sometimes true - some girls do like princesses, some men do like football - these things are not true for all men and all girls.

Also point out that since we now know that gender is a spectrum, it makes these stereotypes seem even more untrue.

Watch Video: "Run Like a Girl"

You might introduce the video this way: *We're going to watch a video about how some of these stereotypes can be harmful to girls and women. Let's watch this video about the stereotypes many of us still have - in this case, about what it means to do something "like a girl."*

Prepare to show the video, being careful to choose your starting point to skip YouTube ads: https://youtu.be/XjJQBjWYDTs

Play the video and STOP the video at 00:39

> *NOTE: This might be a good moment to take a quick Mindful Moment - just three deep breaths - before moving on. You can call for a Mindful Moment anytime you feel the class needs to settle before continuing with the discussion.*

Discuss

- What do you think about this?
- Did you notice that everybody did basically the same thing when they were asked to run or throw or fight like a girl?
- Where do you think these ideas or stereotypes come from?

Resume the video and STOP it again at 1:09

Discuss

- Why do you think the little girls had a different response to the question "What does it mean to run like a girl?"
- How does it make you feel to see the answers of the little girls?

Resume the video and watch until the end.

Discuss

- Where do you think the idea of doing something "like a girl" came from?

- Why is it still a common bias even though we have lots of examples of amazing women athletes like Serena Williams and Megan Rapinoe?

- Do you think that the people who were asked to "run like a girl" thought that they were biased against girls?

- What would it sound like to you if I said that somebody "did math like a girl" or "wrote an essay like a girl?"

- How do you think taking time to think about and notice our thoughts could be helpful in understanding these stereotypes about girls?

- Do you agree with the video that it is possible to change a stereotype like "like a girl" and turn it into something positive?

Peace Partners

Give students time to share what they did for the Peace Partners.

Assign new Peace Partners. Remind your students that their job is to do at least one kind thing for their Peace Partner this week.

Closing words: *Okay, our time is up for today. Thank you for a great class, everyone.*

Optional: *Let's have a nice quiet moment for the bell. If you want to, you can close your eyes, picture your new Peace Partner, and imagine yourself doing something kind for them this week.*

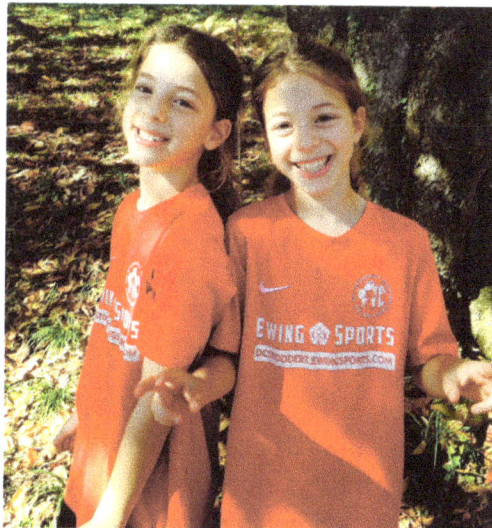

Lesson 23
Everybody Cries

OBJECTIVES: Explore stereotypes and bias

Engage students in mindfulness

Establish terms

Practice kindness

Assign new Peace Partners

PREPARATION: Review lesson

Your Peace Partners list

Prepare to show the videos, being careful to choose your starting point to skip YouTube ads on the second one:

https://www.youtube.com/watch?v=G3Aweo-74kY
A Class That Turned Around Kids' Assumptions of Gender Roles! *Upworthy*

https://www.youtube.com/watch?v=aTvGSstKd5Y
"Boys and Girls on Stereotypes" from *NY Magazine* Series "How to Raise a Boy"

Optional: bell or chime

Optional: student journals

In this lesson we'll be talking again about gender stereotypes and why gender bias can be harmful. In the previous lesson, we focused on stereotypes associated with girls. Today we'll watch two videos in which kids talk about gender stereotypes and what it means to be a boy or a girl in our society and discuss the implications of holding and acting on these stereotypes.

Recommended reading: please see Lesson 22

Introduction

You might say: *In this lesson we'll be talking about gender stereotypes and why gender bias can be harmful to everyone. Today we'll watch two videos in which kids talk about gender stereotypes and what it means to be a boy or a girl in our society. We'll start with Remote Control Breathing again today. As* *always this is optional. If you want to sit quietly and think about something else that is always your choice.*

Mindfulness Practice

Invite today's Mindfulness Leader(s) (ML) to come to the front of the class.

Prompt the ML to say: "Let's sit up a little straighter. Close your eyes or look down into your lap. Let's take 3 deep breaths."

Repeat *Remote Control Breathing from Lesson 8.*

After a few moments, say: *Now take one more deep breath in and out.*

Optional: Ask ML to ring the bell.

Ask students to open their eyes and/or look up when they are ready.

Cue the ML to return to their seat(s).

Discuss

Take a moment to let students share what they were noticing in their minds today.

You might ask:

- Did your mind's remote control change the channel?
- What did you end up "watching?"
- Were you able to change the channel back to the "Breathing Channel?"

Say: *We are going to keep practicing remote control breathing. When it is easier for us to notice what we are thinking in general, it becomes easier to notice what we are thinking about ourselves and other people in any given moment.*

Watch two videos on stereotypes

Say: *Today we are going to watch two videos about gender stereotypes. Can anybody remind us what that means?*

Take a few answers.

Watch Video 1: The impact of stereotypes

Say: *In this first video we are going to explore where some of these stereotypes come from and how common they are.*

https://www.youtube.com/watch?v=G3Aweo-74kY

Discuss

1. What stereotypes did you notice in the video?
2. Why did the kids assume that all of the jobs were held by men?
3. Where do we get these ideas?
4. What impact do you think they might have?

Watch Video 2: Boys and Girls on Stereotypes

Say: *Now we're going to watch a video in which kids talk about what it means to be a boy or a girl in our country. As you listen to them you might think about what we learned about stereotypes in the last lesson and also about the gender spectrum.*

https://www.youtube.com/watch?v=aTvGSstKd5Y "Boys and Girls on Stereotypes"

Discuss

1. What are some of the stereotypes about boys that the kids in the video point out?
2. Can you think of some others that they didn't mention?
3. How do you think these stereotypes could be harmful to boys and men?
4. A lot of the kids in the video mentioned that boys are supposed to be strong and not cry. Do you think it's fair to tell boys that they shouldn't be experiencing or expressing the full range of emotions and feelings that girls are allowed to feel and express?
5. Have you ever felt like these stereotypes have prevented you from being yourself?
6. How do you think these stereotypes could be harmful to people who are non-binary or don't identify as male or female?

> *NOTE: This might be a good moment to take a quick Mindful Moment - just three deep breaths - before moving on.*

Takeaway: Gender Stereotypes Hurt Us All

You might say: *Sometimes people are treated badly, bullied or discriminated against because they don't fit into the gender stereotypes we have about how people <u>should</u> act.*

If men or boys act in a way that is considered to be stereotypically "feminine," then they might be bullied or teased. They might be called "gay." Being gay, or homosexual, just means that you are attracted to people of the same sex as you. It doesn't mean that you act or look a certain way. All straight (heterosexual) people don't act or look the same either.

Gender stereotypes can cause bias. Bias can lead to harmful actions. Here's an example: If you observe someone acting differently from the stereotype you have about that person - maybe you see a boy knitting while other boys play basketball - it can make you feel uncomfortable. It might not seem right because the stereotype you have about boys makes you think that boys shouldn't be knitting. It might even make it seem ok to bully that person, to call them names, for not "acting like a boy should act."

But actually, some boys like to knit. It is important that all people are allowed to express who they really are. **It is never okay to tease, bully or discriminate against someone because of their gender identity, gender expression or sexual orientation.**

Stereotypes and Power

In the United States, men have traditionally held the most power. Women were not given the right to vote until 1920. They were granted this right by men, since men still held all of the power to make laws. Black women, though, faced discrimination that made it extremely hard for them exercise the right to vote until the passage of the Voting Rights Act of 1965. This act prohibited racial discrimination in voting.

People who are transgender, non-binary, homosexual, or on the gender spectrum are still discriminated against in our society. These stereotypes that we have been talking about can help people in power to continue to discriminate against them. It is very important that we learn about this and do what we can to challenge these stereotypes whenever we see or hear them. We'll talk more about how to do this in a later lesson.

Discuss:

- What do you think?
- Can you think of examples of how these gender stereotypes hurt all of us?

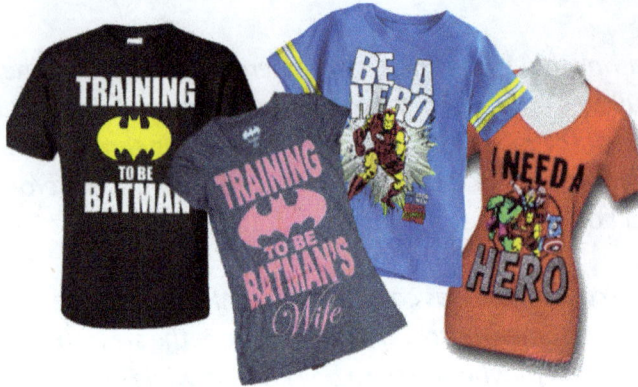

Peace Partners

Give students time to share what they did for the Peace Partners.

Assign new Peace Partners. Remind your students that their job is to do at least one kind thing for their Peace Partner this week.

Closing words: *Okay, our time is up for today. Thank you for a great class, everyone.*

Optional: *Let's have a nice quiet moment for the bell. If you want to, you can close your eyes, picture your new Peace Partner, and imagine yourself doing something kind for them this week.*

Lesson 24
Bias and Discrimination

OBJECTIVES: Continue to explore bias and stereotypes

Engage students in mindfulness

Practice kindness

Assign new Peace Partners

PREPARATION: Review lesson

Prepare to watch this video featuring kids talking about being biracial, racial identity and stereotypes. "Because I'm Latino, I can't have money?" Kids on Race from WNYC's Being 12 Series. https://www.youtube.com/watch?v=C6xSyRJqle8&feature=youtu.be

Your Peace Partners list

Optional: bell or chime

Optional: student journals

Today we will be exploring bias further, looking at how stereotypes lead to bias, and bias leads to discrimination based on race and other factors. Try to listen deeply to your students and their stories today. Remember to remind your students that feeling guilty is normal but not really helpful.

Whenever you need it, before, during or after class, remember you can always Take Five (or do another mindfulness practice). Notice we said "during" class. If you need a moment, take it. If you all need a moment, take it together. If at any time you feel like the discussion is getting heated or feelings are getting intense, you might want to stop and have the class take a few deep breaths. It can be helpful to get more connected to the present moment, to get out of our thoughts for a while, and let things settle before moving on.

Recommended reading: Talking about race and racism is challenging and can bring up a lot of strong emotions. Read these articles to help you to lay some groundwork for the rest of this unit and think about how to respond to what might come up in your discussions.

1. <u>Uncomfortable Conversations with a Black Man</u> In this video series, former NFL linebacker Emmanuel Acho's "sits down to have an "uncomfortable conversation" with white America, in order to educate and inform on racism, system racism, social injustice, rioting & the hurt African Americans are feeling today."

2. <u>Helping Students Discuss Race Openly - Educational Leadership</u> by Julie Landsman.

3. Liz Kleinrock received Teaching Tolerance's 2018 Award for Excellence in Teaching. <u>How to talk about Taboo Subjects with Young Students</u>.

4. From the Anti-Defamation League: <u>How Should I Talk about Race in My Mostly White Classroom</u>?

5. This essay from Peggy McIntosh helps us understand what white privilege is. <u>White Privilege: Unpacking the Invisible Knapsack</u>

6. You will find additional resources in Section VIII: Social Justice Resources.

Introduction

You might say*: Today we are going to be thinking about stereotypes and how they can lead to bias and discrimination against people based on their appearance, their clothes, their religion, and so on. We'll be watching a video in which kids your age talk about their racial identity and how they are treated based on it. We're going to think about how we have experienced bias or discrimination in our own lives.*

First, though, we'll do our remote control breathing mindfulness practice. Mindfulness can really help us consider our thoughts and decide which ones to believe, and which ones to change.

Mindfulness Practice

Invite today's Mindfulness Leader(s) (ML) to come to the front of the class.

Prompt the ML to say: "Let's sit up a little straighter. Close your eyes or look down into your lap. Let's take 3 deep breaths."

Say: *Now let your breath settle back into its natural rhythm. Just breathe. Put your hand on your belly to help you to focus on your breath.*

When you are ready, turn your remote control to the "Counting Your Breaths Channel" and start counting your breaths. Then just try to notice if your mind changes the channel and change it back. You might have to do this over and over. That's perfectly fine. Whenever you notice that your mind has changed the channel you might make a little gesture like you are changing the channel back.

Wait about a minute or so (or longer if it seems like they are able to do more) and then say: *Now you can just let your mind be free to think or not think.*

After a few moments, say: *Now take one more deep breath in and out.*

Optional: Ask ML to ring the bell.

Ask students to open their eyes and/or look up when they are ready.

Cue the ML to return to their seat(s).

Discuss and reflect: What is discrimination?

Ask: Have you ever felt like someone was treated badly because of a stereo-type about someone who looks like you?

Take some answers.

You might say:

When people act on their biases in an unjust way, this is called **discrimination.** *For example:*

- If I as a teacher expect some of my students to do worse at math because of the way they look, I am discriminating against them.
- When a woman isn't paid as much as a man to do the same job, then that woman is being discriminated against.
- The enslavement of African people is an extreme example of discrimination based on racism.

It's really important for us to notice our biases so that we can check to see if we are treating people badly because of them -- without even realizing it.

Racism is discrimination by one person against another person or group of people based on that person or group's "racialized identity" - the race that people think they are by looking at them. Racism can also be "systemic," reflected in the way people of a certain race are treated by society's institutions (schools, courts, businesses and so on). We'll talk more about this after the video.

> *NOTE: This might be a good moment to take a quick Mindful Moment - just three deep breaths - before moving on.*

Now we're going to watch a video that features some students at a school in New York City talking about how they and others are treated based on their skin color, racialized identity, or ethnic identity.

Watch the video <u>"Because I'm Latino, I can't have money?" Kids on Race</u>
https://www.youtube.com/watch?v=C6xSyRJqle8&feature=youtu.be

Prompt the students to notice while they watch:

- Which of these stereotypes have you heard before?
- Which ones have you heard people in your family or community say?
- Which ones have you heard or seen on tv or in movies?
- Have you heard anyone say these things about you?

After the video, ask:

- What examples of bias did you hear in this video?
- Where do you think some of these biases come from? The news? The media?
- Which ones did you find the most surprising to hear?
- Could you relate to what any of these kids was saying?
- Did you hear examples of discrimination in this video? Did the kids who were calling the boys from Ecuador "Mexican" know what they were doing? Is teasing someone about what they eat or about their mother's job discrimination?

> *NOTE: This might be a good moment to take a quick Mindful Moment - just three deep breaths - before moving on.*

Discuss and Reflect: What is white privilege?

You might say: *A white girl in the video referred to "white privilege." Let's go back and listen to that again.*

Go back to the video and play it from 2:24 until she is finished.

Ask the students:

- What do you think about what she says?
- Have you ever noticed that most of the people on tv or in movies are white?
- Have you ever noticed that Band-aids are all "flesh-colored" but there is usually only one color and it matches the skin of most white people?
- Do you think that white privilege, which is also sometimes called white advantage, means that white people are always rich and never struggle? (No, it means that while white people can be poor and face great adversity in life, their struggles are not a result of their skin color.)

You might say: *Most of the time, white people don't even notice that they have white Privilege because they are so used to whiteness being the norm in this country. Usually in a book, if the main character is not described as being a person of color, then we assume that the person is white. White privilege is the result of discrimination against Black people and other people of color.*

Again, if you are white, it is not your fault that you have this advantage. You didn't ask for it. But it is real. It is up to all of us who are white people to recognize this privilege and then to think about what we can do to be anti-racist.

Peace Partners

Give students time to share what they did for the Peace Partners.

Assign new Peace Partners. Remind your students that their job is to do at least one kind thing for their Peace Partner this week.

Closing words: Okay, our time is up for today. Thank you for a great class, everyone.

Optional: *Let's have a nice quiet moment for the bell. If you want to, you can close your eyes, picture your new Peace Partner, and imagine yourself doing something kind for them this week.*

NOTE FROM LINDA: *Dear teacher, How are you doing? You have been leading your students through some challenging and important material. This would be a good time to take a moment to check in with yourself: how are you reacting to the material you are teaching? To the discussions you and your students are having? Where are you noticing these reactions in your own body? In your mind? In your heart?*

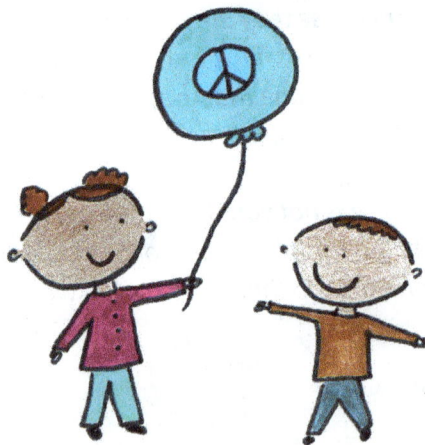

Lesson 25
What is Implicit Bias?

OBJECTIVES: Learn about implicit, or unconscious, bias

Apply knowledge of brain science to help address bias

Engage students in mindfulness

Practice kindness

Assign new Peace Partners

PREPARATION: Review lesson

Your Peace Partners list

Optional: bell or chime

Optional: student journals

In the last lesson we talked discrimination based on conscious bias and prejudice. Today we'll be learning about implicit bias, sometimes called unconscious bias. When it comes to how we think about other people, it is important to try to notice our implicit biases and then decide whether they reflect our values. Mindfulness can help us to notice that our thoughts, including our biases about other people, are just thoughts, not facts. If we can notice that we have biases, we can take some time to decide if we actually believe them or not.

Racist or sexist actions are examples of acting on these biases, either explicit or implicit. These are challenging things to talk about and **it is important to assure our students that recognizing that you have a bias against someone, perhaps because of the way you were raised or the influence of the media, does not make you a racist.**

In her book, *The Person You Mean to Be: How Good People Fight Bias*, social psychologist Dr. Dolly Chugh writes about the need to let go of the "Good Person/Bad Person binary." She argues that it is more productive to see ourselves and others as people who can be in the process of learning at all times, and when we know better, we do better.

"Recognizing our bias doesn't make us racist but it can make us anti-racist."

Dolly Chugh, **author of** *The Person You Mean to Be: How Good People Fight Bias*

We all have biases. Throughout the next few lessons, please communicate to your students that it is important for us to talk about our biases and try to get comfortable with being uncomfortable. Remembering the community agreements you created in Week 1 can help. If we don't recognize and talk about our biases, we can't overcome them.

Background reading: Rhonda Magee offers this helpful explanation for why we teach mindfulness as the foundation for addressing implicit bias. "How Mindfulness Can Defeat Racial Bias". Greater Good Magazine, May 14, 2015.

https://greatergood.berkeley.edu/article/item how_mindfulness_can_defeat_ racial_bias

Introduction

You might say: *Last week we learned about discrimination caused by conscious or explicit bias. Today we'll be learning about something called implicit bias, also called unconscious bias. We all have bias - it's part of being human. What we're here to do is explore what our biases are and decide which ones align with our values and which ones don't. We can see which of our biases aren't helpful and might even be harmful. Mindfulness can help you do this for yourself.*

We'll be practicing mindfulness first and then we'll watch some videos that will help us to notice how we think about other people and whether we are aware of why we think about others in certain ways.

Review Community Agreements:

- Review the Community Agreements from Week 1.
- Identify any agreements you want to revise or reframe.

Mindfulness Practice

Invite today's Mindfulness Leader(s) (ML) to come to the front of the class.

Prompt the ML to say: "Let's sit up a little straighter. Close your eyes or look down into your lap. Let's take 3 deep breaths."

Repeat Remote Control Breathing practice from Lesson 8.

When you notice that your focus has wandered away from your breathing, notice if you are thinking about something that happened in the past or the future, or whether it is about something that is happening right now.

Bring your mind back to your breathing. You might want to try counting your breaths to help you.

After a few moments, say: *Now take one more deep breath in and out.*

Optional: Ask ML to ring the bell.

Ask students to open their eyes and/or look up when they are ready.

Cue the ML to return to their seat(s).

Stereotypes and Bias

You might introduce this lesson by saying: *Let's review what we learned last time about stereotypes. A few lessons ago, we defined stereotypes as "a widely held belief about a group of people that may be true for some of them but is definitely not true for all of them."*

We can also think about stereotypes as our expectations about how people will act based upon the group they belong to. Last week we learned about how stereotypes can make people feel like they must act a certain way based on their gender. We talked about how some people feel that it is ok to bully people who do not conform to gender stereotypes. We talked about how gender stereotypes can be harmful to everyone.

Ask: Did you notice any examples of gender stereotypes this week, maybe even some that you hadn't noticed before?

Take a few answers.

Say: *Today we are going to explore another term: implicit, or unconscious, bias*

You might say: *Sometimes we perceive people as different and have negative feelings about them without even realizing it. This is called implicit or unconscious bias. Everybody has this kind of bias. This bias can come from stereotypes that we hear about from our families or friends, or from commercials we see, or from movies, books, tv shows, and other places.*

Having biases is part of being human.

Sometimes our biases can be a way of protecting us. Do you remember learning about the Negativity Bias? (See Lesson 9) The Negativity Bias is the tendency of our brains to remember bad things that happen to us more than good things; it is a way of keeping us safe. If you burn your hand on a hot stove or a coffee pot your brain will remember that so that you don't do it again. That is a helpful and important bias, most of the time.

Can you think of other ways that your Negativity Bias could help you?

Take a few responses.

Sometimes our Negativity Bias can make us think things that aren't true. What if you get bitten or chased by a dog? Your Negativity Bias might want you to think: "All dogs are dangerous and bad." But that isn't true. It is true that you will get burned if you touch a hot stove, but it is not true that you will get hurt by every dog you meet.

We need to notice that sometimes our Negativity Bias is trying to help us avoid harm when we're not actually in danger. In these situations, the Negativity Bias is not helpful and we need to consciously override the feeling that we are in danger with facts and experiences that counteract it. If we don't, we may take actions that are not in our best interest, or might even be harmful to others.

We can have these same kinds of biases when it comes to people. We noticed in the Gender Stereotypes Lesson that we have a lot of unhelpful or limited ideas about what it means to be a boy or a girl. Most of us don't even notice that we have these biases until they are pointed out to us. When we don't realize we have biases, they are called implicit or unconscious biases.

When it comes to how we think about other people, it is important to try to notice our unconscious biases and then decide whether we agree with what we are thinking.

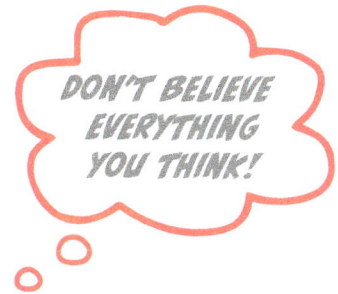

Once we really think about these ideas that we have, we can decide if we want to change them. **Mindfulness helps us to notice that our thoughts and biases are just thoughts, not facts.** If we can notice that we have biases, then we can take some time to decide if we actually believe them or not.

> NOTE: *This might be a good moment to take a quick Mindful Moment - just three deep breaths - before moving on. Use this pause whenever you feel it would be helpful.*

Reflect and Discuss

Share this quote and give a little background about James Baldwin. Baldwin, an African American man, was a famous writer, poet, essayist, playwright, and activist.

> *"Not everything that is faced can be changed, but nothing can be changed until it is faced."*

— James Baldwin

Say: *Before we discuss the quote, I just want to remind us that it is not our fault that we have these unconscious biases or hold these stereotypes in our minds. We didn't choose them and we didn't make them up. We learned them just by watching tv, movies, reading books, playing video games or listening to our friends and family. Most of the time, we don't even realize that we have them.*

Noticing that you have these implicit or unconscious biases does not make you a bad person and does not make you a racist. *But it's important to notice them, or face them, as Baldwin says, so that we can change them if they don't line up with our values.*

Discuss:

- What do you think this quote means?
- What does it mean to "face" things?
- Why can't we change things if we don't face them?
- What does this have to with implicit bias?

Action for the week:

Once again this week, ask students to try to notice any stereotypes that they are aware of, especially ones that they hadn't noticed before. Also ask them to try to notice their own biases.

Peace Partners

Give students time to share what they did for the Peace Partners.

Assign new Peace Partners. Remind your students that their job is to do at least one kind thing for their Peace Partner this week.

Closing words: *Okay, our time is up for today. Thank you for a great class, everyone.*

Optional: *Let's have a nice quiet moment for the bell. If you want to, you can close your eyes, picture your new Peace Partner, and imagine yourself doing something kind for them this week.*

Using Mindfulness to Notice Bias

OBJECTIVE:	Use mindfulness skills to help us notice what we are thinking about others
	Practice kindness
PREPARATION:	Review Body Scan and try it yourself
	Peace Partners List
	Optional: student journals
	Optional: bell or chime

This lesson introduces a method of body scanning that helps students tune into what is happening in their bodies and their feelings. Knowing the language of our bodies can help us determine what kind of response we are having to another person even before we can put words to it. If we can notice it, we can manage it. The Body Scan practice helps students become more familiar with the language of their bodies.

This is a good time to remind your students that they always have a choice about whether to participate in a given mindfulness practice. We hope they will try, but it is always up to them.

As with any lesson in this curriculum, you can use this script to begin, and then and adapt it to make it your own in the future.

Introduction

Say: *Today we are going to learn a type of body scanning called "Flashlight Scanning." During our Mindfulness Practice, I will guide you through the flashlight body scan.*

But first, let's start with this: Put your arms out in front of you with your palms facing each other. Clap your hands together hard and leave your hands about a foot apart. You will notice an intense tingling feeling.

Now, close your eyes, or look down into your lap if you don't feel comfortable closing your eyes, and put your arms out in front of you like I did. When I say 'Go,' clap your hands. Don't talk, but just quietly notice what you feel. Go.

Give them a moment to notice the feelings.

Say: *Open your eyes or look up when you can't feel that tingling anymore.*

Discuss what that felt like.

Mindfulness Practice

Invite today's Mindful Leader(s) (ML) to come to the front of the class.

Prompt the ML to say: "Let's sit up a little straighter. Close your eyes or look down into your lap. Let's take 3 deep breaths."

Say: *Today we are going to be paying attention to our bodies with our minds.*

Take your time with this and talk softly. Remind your students that it's okay if they don't feel anything; the important thing is just to try.

Remind them that you will be asking them questions but that they will be answering the questions in their own minds silently and that we will share later.

Use this script:

Today we are going to do a Flashlight body scan. You can lie down if you feel comfortable doing that; otherwise you may sit in a chair.

Close your eyes and try to make your body so still that the only thing you can feel moving is your breath. Imagine that you have a big flashlight hanging over your body. Imagine that you can operate this flashlight with your mind. Turn it on. Turn it off. Turn it on again.

Move it so that it is shining on your feet. Move it so that it is shining on your head. We're going to use the flashlight to help us to focus on different parts of our bodies.

Start by shining the flashlight on your right foot. Notice if you can feel any sensations there. Is it warm…. cold…. itchy…. Do you feel your sock? Does it feel soft or scratchy? Are your shoes tight or loose?

Now move your flashlight to your left foot. Do you notice any differences? Is it warmer or colder than your right foot? What do you notice?

Now move your flashlight up to your knees. What do you feel there? Can you feel the fabric of your pants or leggings? Can you feel the air on your knees?

Now move your flashlight to your right hand. Can you still feel the tingling feeling from the big clap or has that gone away? Does your hand feel cold or warm, dry or a little sweaty?

Now move your flashlight to your left hand. What is different over there? Is one hand warmer than the other? How does your left hand feel?

Now move your flashlight to your belly. There is always something going on in your belly so it's a good place to notice sensations. Maybe it's almost time for lunch and you can feel that your stomach is empty. Maybe you have just eaten lunch and you can feel your food digesting. Maybe you can feel your belly rising and falling with your breath. Try to notice that for a few breaths.

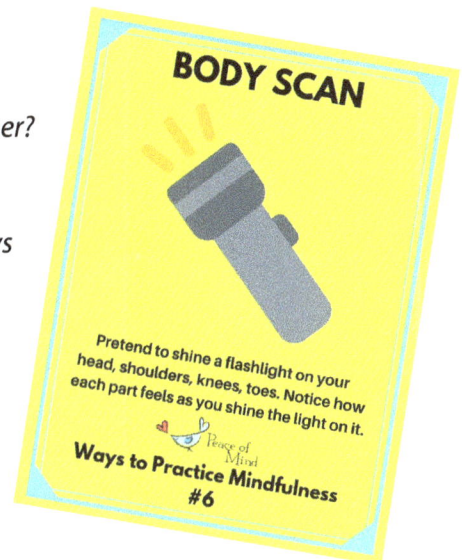

BODY SCAN

Pretend to shine a flashlight on your head, shoulders, knees, toes. Notice how each part feels as you shine the light on it.

Peace of Mind

Ways to Practice Mindfulness #6

Now move your flashlight to your chest. Maybe you can feel your heart beating. Maybe you can feel your chest rising and falling as your lungs fill up with air and empty again. Try to notice that for a few breaths.

Now move your flashlight up to your face. Shine it on your right eye. What do you feel there? What does it feel like to have your eyelid closed? Move it to your other eye? Any differences?

Move your flashlight to your nose. Can you feel the air going in and out? Maybe you can't. Just try to notice it.

Move your flashlight to your mouth. Focus on your tongue. What does it feel like? Is it dry or wet? Is it itchy?

Move your flashlight to your teeth. Can you feel your teeth without touching them with your tongue? If you have braces you definitely know what your teeth feel like when your braces have been tightened. How do you know that you have teeth if you can't see them?

Move your flashlight to the top of your head. Can you feel your hair with your mind?

Now pull your flashlight back so that it is shining on your whole body. What do you notice? Maybe you are feeling really relaxed and could stay here all day. Maybe you are feeling antsy and can't wait to get up. Any way that you feel is fine. Just try to notice what it feels like.

After a few moments, say: *Now take one more deep breath in and out.*

Optional: Ask ML to ring the bell.

Ask students to open their eyes and/or look up when they are ready.

Cue the ML to return to their seat(s).

Reflect and Discuss

- What did it feel like to travel through your body?
- What did you notice?
- Are you used to paying attention to your body?
- Would it be helpful to pay more attention to your body?
- What about when you are playing a sport?
- What about when you are in school?

Guided Reflection:

Say: *Now that you've paid attention to your body, I'm going to lead you in a really short guided reflection. This time we're going to be paying attention to our thoughts and our bodies at the same time. I'm going to ask you to think about some things and then try to notice what your first reaction is and what you notice in your body. Try to be as honest with yourself as possible. You can close your eyes or look down into your lap.*

Okay, try to imagine this:

You are choosing teams for a basketball game. There are two people left - one is a tall girl and one is a heavier but shorter boy. Who do you choose?

Pause for a moment or two.

Try to notice what is happening in your mind and your body.

Okay, now try to imagine this:

You are waiting to be chosen for a team for a basketball game. You and one other person are the only two people waiting to be chosen. The other person is different from you in height, weight, skin color, ability to play basketball. Which one of you do you think will get picked first? How does that make you feel? What do you notice in your body?

Pause for a moment or two.

Take a deep breath and open your eyes if they were closed.

Reflect and Discuss

Invite students to share. Make sure students feel welcome to share but please do not make it mandatory. If you think it would work better for your class, consider letting students write their answers in a journal.

Review Scenario 1: *You are choosing teams for a basketball game at recess. There are two people left - one is a tall girl and one is a heavier but shorter boy. Who do you choose?*

Ask: So what kinds of things came up for you when you were trying to decide? Did you notice any bias?

- Maybe you were thinking - "tall people are better at basketball." Is that a stereotype?
- Maybe you were thinking "girls aren't good at sports." Is that a stereotype?
- Maybe you were thinking that the boy wouldn't be good because he is heavy. Is that a stereotype?
- Maybe you were thinking, "I already have three girls on my team and I should make it more balanced."
- Maybe you were thinking that you felt sorry for one of the kids and wanted to pick them.
- Maybe you were thinking something else.

It might help to say: *Remember, we all have stereotypes, and we all have bias. When we can notice what we are thinking, we can make a decision about whether to believe the stereotype or not. We can control our thoughts.*

Ask: Does anybody want to share some of your reactions?

Take a few responses.

Review Scenario 2: *You are waiting to be chosen for a team for a group project in school. You and one other person are the only two people waiting to be chosen. The other person is different from you in most ways. Which one of you do you think will get picked first?*

What did you notice?

- How were you picturing the other kid?
- What did they look like?
- How did the way they looked determine whether you thought you or they would be picked?
- How did it feel to be the one likely to be picked or the one unlikely to be picked?

Recognizing different types of bias

In your discussion, more than one type of bias will probably come up. Use these descriptions to help students identify different types of bias, including racial bias, gender bias, and body image bias.

Body image bias

You might say: *Another type of bias that we haven't talked about much so far relates to body type. When we look at tv, movies, and commercials, we don't just see a majority of white people, we see a majority of thin people. If you were just watching tv, you would think that the average person was thin or muscular or very fit. Many of the pictures that we see on the internet and in magazines are airbrushed to make the celebrities or models look much thinner than they actually are.*

Ask: Do you think that that stereotype of thinness could make people feel badly about themselves if they don't fit that mold? Do you think that people might discriminate against people who aren't thin?

Racial Bias

You might say: *Did you notice that I didn't mention anything about the race of the two kids? How did you picture the two kids in your mind? Did you picture* *them as white? Our culture is dominated by white people. White people are overwhelmingly represented in tv, movies, books, commercials, billboards, and so on. Because of that, some people just assume that we are talking about white people if no race is mentioned.*

Ask*: Think about how you pictured the two kids. How do you think your own identity affected the way you pictured them?*

Gender Bias – please refer back to Lessons 21 and 22.

Action for the week

Engage your students in further reflection by asking them to notice bias in the time between Peace of Mind classes.

You might say: *This week try to keep a list of examples of bias you notice coming up in your mind as you interact with people or with tv, social media, movies, video games, etc. See if you can notice when you see an example of something that challenges your bias. Write down what you notice in your journal or somewhere else. We'll have time to share what you noticed in our next class.*

Peace Partners

Give students time to share what they did for the Peace Partners.

Assign new Peace Partners. Remind your students that their job is to do at least one kind thing for their Peace Partner this week.

Closing words: *Okay, our time is up for today. Thank you for a great class, everyone.*

Optional*: Let's have a nice quiet moment for the bell. If you want to, you can close your eyes, picture your new Peace Partner, and imagine yourself doing something kind for them this week.*

Lesson 27
That's Not Me!

OBJECTIVES:	Continue to explore bias and stereotypes
	Engage students in mindfulness
	Practice kindness
	Assign new Peace Partners
PREPARATION:	Review lesson
	Your Peace Partners list
	Copies of the Starburst worksheet found at the end of this lesson for each student
	Optional: bell or chime
	Optional: student journals

We have been covering some challenging material. You might want to start this class with a game or an ice-breaker. You could do a round of Count to Ten from Lesson 3 or choose another one of your class favorites.

After mindfulness, we're going to spend today revisiting students' identity maps. Students will have a chance to look back at what they wrote in Lesson 2, if you have those available. They'll then make new "Starburst" identity maps that chart not only how they see themselves, but how they think others see them. Kids usually enjoy this exercise which often leads to new and important insights about themselves and the world around them. You might try to make a Starburst yourself.

Background video: We found this to be a helpful background video for talking about race and racism with students. Take a few minutes to have a look before class. The Myth of Race with Jenée Desmond Harris . https://www.youtube.com/watch?v=VnfKgffCZ7U

Introduction

> **You might say:** *In this lesson we talk more about identity. We look at how who we are doesn't always match how we are viewed by society. We are also going to talk about race and what that really means.*

Mindfulness Practice: Four Square Breathing

Invite today's Mindful Leaders (ML) to come to the front of the class.

Prompt the ML to say: "Let's sit up a little straighter. Close your eyes or look down into your lap. Let's take 3 deep breaths."

Then you might say: *Okay let's try doing Four Square Breathing. We'll do it together. Remember you're just drawing or imaging a square as you breathe in for 4 beats, hold your breath for 4 beats, breathe out for four beats, and wait for four beats.*

Let's try it: Breathe in 1,2,3,4 (count slowly)

> *Hold your Breath 1,2,3,4*
> *Breathe out 1,2,3,4*
> *Wait 1,2,3,4*

Repeat 2 or 3 times

Say: *Take one big deep breath and reach your arms up over your head as you breathe in and slowly float them down as you breathe out.*

Optional: Ask ML to ring the bell.

Ask students to open their eyes and/or look up when they are ready.

Cue the ML to return to their seat(s).

Identity

Say: *Today we are going to work on our Identity Maps again.*

Activity 1. Review Identity Maps

Review Identity Maps from Lesson 2, if possible. Hand out copies of their original identity chart if available.

Students will make new Identity Maps called Starburst Maps.

Ask students to:

1. Write their name in the middle.

2. Fill out aspects of their identity, just like we did in Lesson 2. Write these on the lines with the arrow pointing **away** from their name.

Give them a few minutes to do this. They can be copying from their other Identity Map or starting over.

Ask: *What do you notice about what you included in your Starburst Identity Map? What is missing? There might be things missing that you decided not to share for personal reasons. There might be things you just didn't think of.*

Take some answers.

Ask*: If you are white did you list that as part of your identity? If you are not white, did you list your race as part of your identity? Why or why not?*

Take some answers.

You might say*: Let's talk for a moment about race and racial identity.*

Here are some important ideas and concepts to share and discuss.

White Identity

If you are white you might not have listed that as part of your identity. White people are not usually accustomed to thinking of themselves as white. This concept can even make some white people feel uncomfortable. This might be why you might not have listed being white as part of your identity even if you are considered to be white.

It's important to know that racial categories were created by people. They aren't based in science or genetics. Our physical differences, like skin color, were orig-

inally just the result of where we lived in the world and how we adapted to the conditions we lived in.

Ideas about race have changed over time and vary by country, even in different states in the US. People who were once not considered white, over time came to be considered white. People who are considered white in other countries might not be considered white in this country. People who are considered white can be descended from Irish or Italian or German ancestors or from many other places. Those countries are all very different in language and culture but in this country most people who came from Europe were encouraged to assimilate when they immigrated - to try to all become the same - to become "white."

If you are a person of color, your racialized identity (the race that other people perceive you to be) might seem like a bigger part of your identity because of discrimination, or it might be a source of pride.

Race is an idea

Racial categories are not based in science or genetics. They were made up by people in power in the 1700s and served to defend the institution of enslavement. When those in power in the early days of the United States were able to say that the "White" race was separate from and superior to the "Black" race, they were able to use race to try to justify enslaving African people while building a country based on the ideas of freedom for all men. So being white, like all other racial categories, was an idea that was created for a purpose.

Racism is real

Even though this _idea_ of race is not real, people are treated _very_ differently based on their racialized identity - what race they are considered to be by society. That is what we call racism.

Reflect and Discuss

1. Are you surprised by this idea of race as an idea?

2. This definition of race is based in the modern science of genetics and is different from what many people have been taught. How does this make you feel about race and racism?

3. Are there other aspects of your Starburst Identity Map that you think you might have left out?

Activity 2: Finish the Starburst Identity Map

Say: *Now we are going to add to our Starburst Identity Map. This time we're going to add any labels that are given to us by other people.*

*I want you to think about how **other** people see you. How do people label you?*

You could share these examples:

1. Maybe you are the oldest of four or five children. You might have been given the role of being a caretaker for your younger siblings. You might feel like you are seen as more grown up than you really are.

2. Maybe you are really into sports but since you wear glasses people label you as smart or "nerdy."

3. Maybe you are into music and drawing but since you are tall and strong people label you as someone who loves football and sports.

4. Maybe you love sports and playing video games but since you are a girl people think that you like cooking or taking care of kids and they label you as the babysitter.

5. In the video we watched in the last class, some of the kids talked about how people assume things about them because of the way they look. One girl says that some kids tease another boy about eating tacos because they think he's from Mexico. So that boy might feel that he has been labeled as Mexican even though he is from Ecuador. There is nothing wrong with being Mexican! But it's just not who he is. The kids who are calling him Mexican aren't making the effort to see him as he is.

Ask: Does anybody want to share a label that's been applied to you?

Ask the students to write these kinds of labels given to them by others on the lines that are pointing toward the middle, **toward your name.**

It could be powerful for you to share what your own map would look like. For me, because I have blonde hair I was often called a "dumb blonde" when I was a kid as that was a common stereotype back then. So I might write that on one of the lines going in toward my name. Because other people saw me that way, it affected the way I felt about myself and I lost confidence academically. It was also assumed that I wasn't athletic because I was a girl and there weren't as many opportunities for girls to play sports back in the 1970s.

Share

When they are finished, you can have individual students share or do a gallery walk.

Reflect and Discuss

- What labels do you think other people put on you?
- Where do you think these ideas come from?
- Do any of these labels affect how you feel about yourself?

Peace Partners

Give students time to share what they did for the Peace Partners.

Assign new Peace Partners. Remind your students that their job is to do at least one kind thing for their Peace Partner this week.

Closing words: *Okay, our time is up for today. Thank you for a great class, everyone.*

Optional: *Let's have a nice quiet moment for the bell. If you want to, you can close your eyes, picture your new Peace Partner, and imagine yourself doing something kind for them this week.*

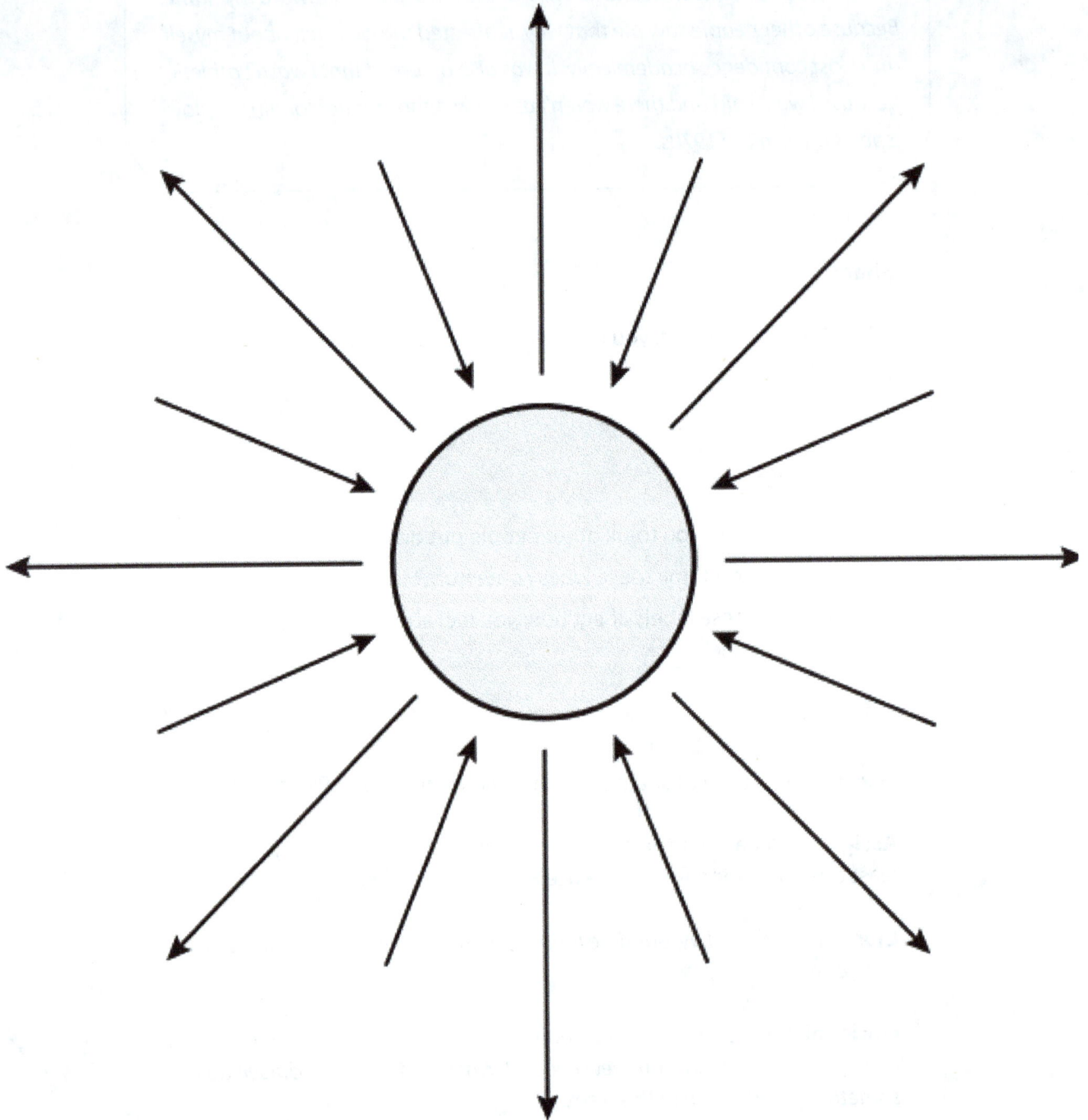

Starburst Worksheet

Lesson 28
Counter Stereotypes

OBJECTIVE: Use mindfulness skills to help us notice what we are thinking about others

Practice kindness

PREPARATION: Review Lesson

Your Peace Partners list

Optional: bell or chime

Optional: student journals

In the last few lessons, we have seen how stereotypes can lead to bias and discrimination. Perhaps your conversations have already moved to action: what can we do about this? In this lesson, you will be able to explore the importance of counter stereotypes with your students, and give them the opportunity to create a collage that refutes the harmful stereotypical images we often see in the media.

Teacher Resource: This Nick News segment on Black Lives Matter is good background for the conversations you may be having today. *Kids, Race and Unity hosted by Alicia Keys* https://www.youtube.com/watch?v=OWsMEIODo6g

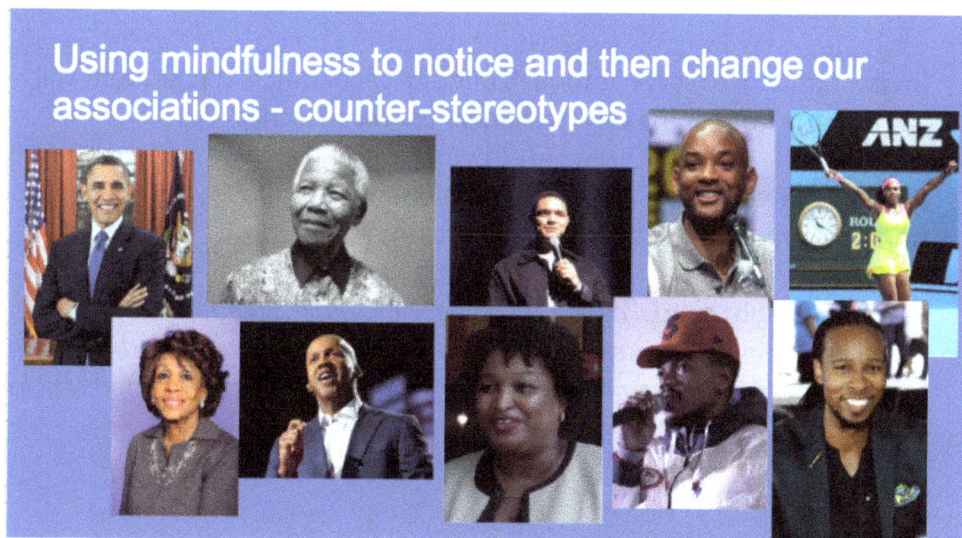

Pictured from top left: Barack Obama, Nelson Mandela, Trevor Noah, Will Smith, Serena Williams, Representative Maxine Waters, Bryan Stevenson, Stacy Abrams, Chance the Rapper, Dr. Ibram X Kendi

Introduce Lesson

You might say: *So far we have seen how stereotypes about people can lead to bias and discrimination. What can we do about it?*

When we see stereotypes over and over, they start to become more real in our minds, even though they aren't actually true. The movie Hidden Figures tells the story of Black women who were mathematicians who worked for NASA and helped to put the first astronauts on the moon. This movie is important because it is an opportunity for Black girls and all girls to see women in roles that disprove common stereotypes. It also reveals how much discrimination the women in the movie faced as they tried to do their work.

It's important to remember that people of color and women got stuck in stereo-typical roles in society -- like housewife, nurse, teacher, maid-- not because those were the only jobs that they wanted, but because those were the only jobs that the people who were in charge of companies and institutions allowed them to have.

Today you will have an opportunity to think about how stereotypes affect you personally, and then you will create a collage, a song, a poem or another creation that shows examples of people who are the opposite of a stereotype – a counter-stereotype. But first, let's get settled in with 4 Square Breathing.

Mindfulness Practice

Invite a student to serve as today's Mindful Leader(ML). This student will come to the front of the class to sit next to you on a chair.

Prompt the ML to say: "Let's sit up a little straighter. Close your eyes or look down into your lap. Let's take 3 deep breaths."

Then you might say: *Okay let's try doing Four Square Breathing. We'll do it together. Remember you're just drawing or imaging a square as you breathe in for 4 beats, hold your breath for 4 beats, breathe out for four beats, and wait for four beats.*

Let's try it: Breathe in 1,2,3,4 (count slowly)

Hold your Breath 1,2,3,4
Breathe out 1,2,3,4
Wait 1,2,3,4

Repeat 2 or 3 times

Say: *Okay, great job! Let's take one big deep breath and reach your arms up over your head as you breathe in and slowly float them down as you breathe out.*

Optional: Ask ML to ring the bell.

Ask students to open their eyes and/or look up when they are ready.

Cue the ML to return to their seat(s).

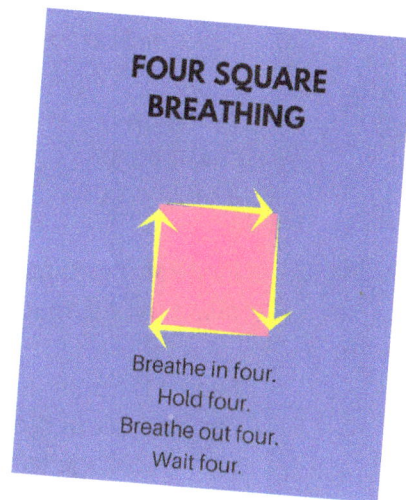

How do stereotypes affect me?

Following are two activities to help students reflect on how stereotypes affect them personally.

1. **Recording Stereotypes**

   Ask each student to write on a strip of paper about a stereotype that has been applied to them and why the stereotype doesn't fit. No names required.

   Post all of the strips anonymously, inviting students to think about how stereotypes make their classmates feel.

   Discuss

   • What did you notice about what your classmates shared?
   • Were you surprised by what you read?
   • Did you see examples of stereotypes that you weren't aware of before?

2. **Counter Stereotype Project**

   Each student will create a counter-stereotype collage, drawing, poem, rap, song, or a combination - This can also be done with a partner or in a small group.

   Invite students to focus on one stereotype. It can be one that they can relate to personally or not.

   Search for examples of people who **do not** represent that stereotype. For example: If the stereotype is that girls aren't athletic, you could make a collage featuring Serena Williams, Megan Rapinoe, etc.

   Invite students to reflect back on the second version of their Identity Maps.

   Invite them to consider what they can add to their project that celebrates what is special about them and/or people who have similar identities to theirs.

   What would they want to tell people in order to counter a stereotype about themselves or about other people that is not fair?

   When students are finished, consider posting projects around the room and having a gallery walk.

Peace Partners

   Give students time to share what they did for the Peace Partners.

   Assign new Peace Partners. Remind your students that their job is to do at least one kind thing for their Peace Partner this week.

   Closing words: Okay, our time is up for today. Thank you for a great class, everyone.

   Optional: *Let's have a nice quiet moment for the bell. If you want to, you can close your eyes, picture your new Peace Partner, and imagine yourself doing something kind for them this week.*

Lesson 29
Practice Speaking Up

OBJECTIVE: Explore how to use what we have learned to stand
up against unfair and unkind treatment of another.

Practice kindness

PREPARATION: Review Lesson

Your Peace Partners list

5 copies of the *Speaking Up* skit found at end of
lesson, if needed

Optional: bell or chime

Optional: student journals

Today we move into a discussion of the most important and challenging
choices a young person can make: to stand up for someone who is being
bullied or discriminated against. Today we'll address this in mindfulness practice, through a skit and through a story. There are a few different choices of
activities. Choose the ones that you think will be most appropriate for your
students.

Background Reading: We recognize no two communities will be facing the
same set of challenges. This handbook from Teaching Tolerance can help you
frame possible responses to the particular issues facing your school and your
students. https://www.tolerance.org/sites/default/files/general/speak_up_
handbook.pdf

Introduction

Say: *Now we are going to start thinking about standing up for ourselves and
others. We're going to start out with a guided reflection. In this practice, I am
going to describe some things that might happen in school or somewhere else.
I am going to ask you where you feel your reactions in your body.*

Mindfulness Practice

Invite the Mindful Leader(s) (ML) to come to the front of the class to sit next to you on a chair.

Prompt the ML to say: "Let's sit up a little straighter. You may choose to close your eyes or look down into your lap. Let's take 3 deep breaths."

Then you say: *I'm going to describe a few different situations and I'd like you to imagine that they are happening to you. Try to notice how you feel and where in your body you feel it.*

- Imagine that you are hanging out with a few kids at the park, and somebody runs up and says something mean to your friend. Everybody except your friend laughs at what he says, including you. How do you feel? Where do you feel it?

- Now imagine that you are hanging out with a few kids at the park, and somebody runs up and says something mean to your friend. The other kids laugh, but you don't. You walk over to your friend and say "Let's get out of here." How do you feel? Where do you feel it?

- Imagine that you are hanging out with a few kids at the park and somebody runs up and says something mean to you. Everybody laughs except for you. How do you feel? Where do you feel it?

- Now imagine that you are hanging out with a few kids at the park and somebody runs up and says something mean to you. Everybody laughs except for one person. She comes over to you and says, "Let's get out of here." How do you feel? Where do you feel it?

- Imagine you are outside at the park and you run up to some kids and you say something mean to one of them. Everybody laughs except for the person you were mean to. How do you feel? Where do you feel it?

- Imagine you are outside at the park and you run up to some kids and you say something mean to one of them. Nobody laughs. How do you feel? Where do you feel it?

Invite students to take three deep breaths.

Optional: Ask ML to ring the bell.

Ask students to open their eyes and/or look up when they are ready.

Cue the ML to return to their seat(s).

Reflect and Discuss

Ask: *Does anybody want to share what you were feeling or thinking about*?

Replay each situation and ask for people to share how they felt in different situations.

Ask:

- Why might you laugh when someone says something mean, even if you don't think it's funny or you feel sorry for the person getting teased?
- How did it feel when you were the one saying something mean and everybody laughed?
- What did it feel like when nobody laughed?
- How did you feel when you said to your friend "Let's get out of here?

Point out how our approval or disapproval can "train" people to keep doing things or stop doing things.

Talk about how powerful it can be to stand there and not laugh.

Talk about how there is no such thing as a neutral bystander. You are either helping the target of the bullying or unkindness or you are helping the person doing the bullying or unkindness. Your silence will be interpreted as agreement with the mean words or actions. Unless you say something to help the person being harmed you are helping to harm them.

Speaking Up

Choose from one of the following approaches

1. Students act out the *Speaking Up* skit
2. Students read the *Speaking Up* skit aloud from their seats
3. Teacher reads the skit aloud and class discusses

For options 1 and 2, choose 5 actors to play Lyle, Shonda, Crystal, Damien and Dex.

Hand out copies of the skit and have them act it out or read it.

Instruct the audience to notice what they feel in their bodies as the skit plays out and think about what they would have done in this situation.

Act/Read/Listen to the skit.

Reflect and Discuss

- Why is it important to say something?
- What are you saying if you remain silent?
- What were Crystal's friends saying to her by going along when she was bullying the younger kids?
- Did they use words or actions to say something to Crystal by the end of the story?
- What would you have said if you were Dex or Damien?

Peace Partners

Give students time to share what they did for the Peace Partners.

Assign new Peace Partners. Remind your students that their job is to do at least one kind thing for their Peace Partner this week.

Closing words: *Okay, our time is up for today. Thank you for a great class, everyone.*

Optional: *Let's have a nice quiet moment for the bell. If you want to, you can close your eyes, picture your new Peace Partner, and imagine yourself doing something kind for them this week.*

Lesson 29
Speaking Up Skit

Topic: Speaking Up

Scene: 6th graders Lyle and Shonda are waiting for the bus after school

Characters: Lyle, Shonda, Crystal, Dex, Damien

_____

Lyle: That concert we heard today was really cool!

Shonda: Yeah, I thought the drumline was awesome.

Lyle: Thanks for waiting for the bus with me.

Shonda: No problem.

8th graders Crystal, Dex and Damien walk in.

Lyle: Oh no! Here comes Crystal and her friends again. Why can't they leave me alone?

Shonda: What do you mean?

Lyle: They bother me every day. They are always teasing me about something. It's awful.

Dex: I thought we were going to miss the bus. Everybody was so slow on the stairs.

Crystal: (*pointing at Lyle and Shonda*) Oh, look at the little babies at the bus stop. Let's go say Hello!

Damien: Oh Crystal, don't bother those kids again..

Crystal: (*to Lyle and Shonda*) Hello babies! How's life in Pre-K?

Lyle and Shonda look uncomfortable and try to ignore her

Crystal: (*looks at Lyle's shoes*) OMG! What are you wearing? Guys, look at his ratty old sneakers!

Damien: (looking at his own shoes) They look better than mine.

Crystal: Are you kidding? They're disgusting!

Dex and Damien look at each other and look uncomfortable.

Crystal: (*laughing in a mean way*) I bet all of your shoes are hand me downs.

Lyle covers his face and looks like he's about to cry. Shonda looks down at her hands.

Dex: Hey Crystal, why don't you leave them alone?

Crystal: What do you mean?

Damien: It's just not funny anymore.

Crystal: If you don't think it's funny, why don't you go join the babies?

Dex: I think I will! (*Moves to sit with Lyle and Shonda*). Hey guys, wasn't that drumline cool today?

Damien: (*he sees what Dex is doing and decides to do it too*) Oh yeah, I love those drums! I think I'm going to try out.

Lyle and Shonda smile.

Crystal is suddenly alone and looks uncomfortable and unhappy.

Crystal: Come on guys, you don't want to hang out with those kindergarten babies. Let's go..

(Dex and Damien ignore her)

Crystal: Oh whatever. I'm out of here. (*Crystal walks out*)

Lyle: Thanks you guys.

Dex: No problem!

All smile.

The End

Lesson 30
Burgers and Bullying

OBJECTIVES:

Help us to take action when we witness or experience unkind action based on bias

Recognize the powerful role a bystander can play in stopping bullying

Help to build the courage to stand up for ourselves and others.

Engage students in mindfulness

Practice kindness

Assign new Peace Partners

PREPARATION:

Review lesson

Your Peace Partners list

Burger King video. Make sure to prepare the video so that you skip any YouTube ads: https://www.youtube.com/watch?v=mnKPEsbTo9s&feature=youtu.be[5]

6 copies of the *Dude* skit, if needed, found at end of lesson

Optional: bell or chime

Optional: student journals

In this lesson we'll be learning about another way of standing up for someone and interrupting bias. We'll be watching a video showing how sometimes people do not stand up for others and why sometimes they do. There is also the option to act out a skit that gives students an option to say "dude!" when they want to say something when someone is being bullied or mistreated. It might seem funny to them to use that word and that is part of the fun. This should be used as a jumping off point, a way to encourage them to start to say something when they see injustice or mean behavior. If "dude" is not relevant to your kids, by all means have them brainstorm words that they might be more likely to use.

---

5   Today the lesson includes a video made by a fast food company. We are in no way endorsing the company, nor do we have any relationship with the company of any kind.

> **NOTE FROM LINDA:** *I always find that kids are nervous about tattling. I tell them that the difference between tattling and telling is their motivation. If you are trying to get someone in trouble you are tattling. If you are trying to help someone who's in trouble you are telling.*

Introduction

Say: *Today we are going to explore a little more the idea of what you can do when you see someone being treated unkindly. To help us, we'll be acting out a skit.*

But first, let's do our mindfulness practice.

Mindfulness Practice

Say: *Today we're going to do See, Hear, Feel again but we're going to do it a little differently. We'll do it the usual way first and then we'll do it with a partner. For now, sit next to your Peace Partner. When we get to the partner practice this is how it will work:*

Decide who will go first. Sit in your mindful bodies, eyes closed or down, facing each other. The person who is going first will notice whether they are more aware of see, hear, or feel in that moment and they will say out loud "see", "hear", or "feel."

The other person will notice if they are more aware of see, hear, or feel and will say out loud "see", "hear", or "feel." You'll keep trading off for a few minutes.

Say: *It may be distracting to hear the other people saying "see, hear, or feel." See if you can really pay attention to your partner and to what you are noticing.*

It's fine if you keep saying "Hear" because all you are paying attention to are the sounds of the other people. Just try to notice what is most noticeable for you. You might have an itch or your foot is asleep and so "feel" would be the most noticeable thing.

Don't stress about this - just try to do it with a sense of humor and relax.

Invite the Mindful Leader(s) (ML) to come to the front of the class.

Prompt the ML to say: "Let's sit up a little straighter. Close your eyes or look down into your lap. Let's take 3 deep breaths."

Then you might say: *Okay, so first we're going to do it on our own. So remember, all I am going to say is See, Hear or Feel. You're going to try to move your attention around to focus on those things that you see, hear and feel. Don't worry if you get distracted and start thinking about something else. That's totally normal. As soon as you notice that your mind went somewhere else just try to start again. This might happen a bunch of times and that's fine.*

See... wait about ten seconds

Hear.... wait about ten seconds

Feel.... wait about ten seconds

Repeat this two or three times - if the students seem restless cut it shorter.

Say: *Okay, great job!*

You can open your eyes. Now let's try this with a partner. Turn to your Peace Partner and sit facing them close together. Here's how it works again:

Decide who will go first. Sit in your mindful bodies, eyes closed or down, facing each other. The person who is going first will notice whether they are more aware of see, hear, or feel in that moment and they will say out loud "see", "hear", or "feel."

The other person will notice if they are more aware of see, hear, or feel and will say out loud "see", "hear", or "feel." You'll keep trading off for a few minutes.

Okay, are you ready to try it?

Give them time to get ready with their partner, decide who goes first, etc.

Okay, go!

Wait a minute or two and then say:

Okay, great job! Let's take one big deep breath and reach your arms up over your head as you breathe in and slowly float them down as you breathe out.

Optional: Ask ML to ring the bell.

Cue students to open their eyes and/or look up when they are ready.

Cue the ML to return to their seat(s).

Ask: What did it feel like to do See, Hear, Feel with a partner?

Watch Video

Say: *Today we're going to watch a video about bullying and bias and saying something. This is a video that was made by the Burger King company to show how hard it can be for people to stand up for others.*

Watch the Burger King Bullying video, taking care to set it up to avoid the YouTube ads: https://www.youtube.com/watch?v=mnKPEsbTo9s&feature=youtu.be

Discuss

- Why do you think people were more likely to say something about a smashed cheeseburger than to say something about a kid being bullied?
- What did the people watching look like while the kid was being bullied?
- Who were they helping with their silence?
- What did the people who stood up for the boy being bullied do? Did they get into a fight with the other kids?
- Do you see any similarities between this video and the skit and/or the story that we thought about last time?

Say: *Standing up for other people is hard. Like the boy in the video said, "It's easier to do nothing." But saying something gets easier with practice, and it is easier if you don't do it alone. Today we're going to practice and see what we would or could do in different situations.*

Practice standing up for others

Try role playing a few different ways of handling the problem. If your students aren't comfortable with role playing, you can just read the scenarios and have them discuss options.

1. Four kids are sitting at a lunch table. Someone walks up and asks to join them and someone at the table says "No. Go away Loser!" What can the other kids say or do? (get up and offer to sit with the kid somewhere else; say "Dude!" to the kid who was mean and offer the other kid a spot at the table next to you…)

2. Four kids are on the bus going home. One kid drops her backpack and her stuff spills out all over the bus floor. One kid laughs and points and says "What a klutz!" What can the other kids say or do? (Get up and help the kid pick up her stuff; say "Hey that's not cool.")

3. Two kids are on the school computers. One kid writes something mean about another. What can the other kid do or say?

4. Two girls in class have been bickering for the past couple of weeks. At night, you're on Instagram and you see one of the girls started a new account. However, when you get to her profile, you notice the pictures and comments are not right and actually say mean things about the girl whose account it says it is. You realize that it's a fake account. You see that other classmates are posting disrespectful comments on the pictures and some are probably unaware it's a fake account. What can you do or say?

Ask your students to come up with more scenarios to discuss.

The *Dude* Skit

Acting out or reading through this skit is another way students can practice standing up for others. Choose from one of the following approaches:

1. Students act out the Dude skit.
2. Students read the Dude skit aloud from their seats.
3. Teacher reads the Dude skit aloud.

Note: if your students would rather substitute a more relevant word for "Dude," that's great.

Say: *Today we are going to be [acting out / reading/ listening to] a skit. In this skit some kids are standing up for someone on the playground. Sometimes it is hard to think of the right words to say when you want to help someone. In this skit the kids are all using one helping word. If this word sounds funny or awkward to you, try to think of a word like this that you might use that would have a similar effect.*

In this skit called "Dude" there are 6 kids: Richard, Benson, Aniyah, Andrew, Kidus, and Emmanuel. We need 6 volunteers to act out this skit.

The audience has an important role here. As you hear the characters talk to each other, notice how your body feels. Notice if you have felt any of these feelings before in a similar situation.

For options 1 and 2, choose 6 actors to play Richard, Benson, Aniyah, Andrew, Kidus, Emmanuel. **Hand out** copies of the skit and have them act it out or read it.

Instruct the audience to notice what they feel in their bodies as the skit plays out and think about what they would have done in this situation.

Act out / Read / Listen to the skit.

Discuss

- What do you think of the way the kids handled this situation?
- Did you notice any feelings in your body during the skit?
- Why do you think the word "Dude" was helpful here?
- Is there another word or phrase that you might use instead?
- Have you ever watched a bullying situation when you couldn't think of what to say? it can be hard to think of the right thing. Do you think saying something like "Dude" would be easier?
- Have you seen bullying in tv, movies or books? How have you noticed kids handling it? What have you noticed that works and doesn't work?

Peace Partners

Give students time to share what they did for the Peace Partners.

Assign new Peace Partners. Remind your students that their job is to do at least one kind thing for their Peace Partner this week.

Closing words: *Okay, our time is up for today. Thank you for a great class, everyone.*

Optional: *Let's have a nice quiet moment for the bell. If you want to, you can close your eyes, picture your new Peace Partner, and imagine yourself doing something kind for them this week.*

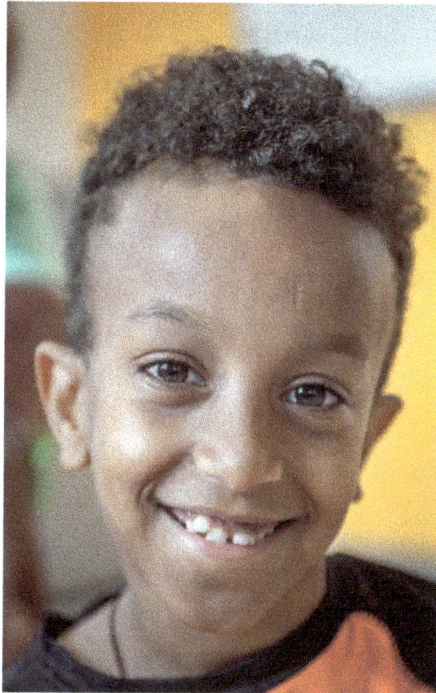

Lesson 30 Skit
Dude: Standing Up for Others

NOTE: *If it makes more sense to substitute another word for "Dude" that is more relevant to your students, please do.*

Topic: Standing up against bullying

Characters: 6 kids: Richard, Benson, Aniyah, Andrew, Kidus and Emmanuel

Setting: A park **or** the playground at recess

_____

Richard: Hey, you guys, let's make some teams for basketball!

Benson: Yeah. I'll be a captain.

Aniyah: I'll be one too.

Andrew: Why do we need captains? Why don't we just count off?

Kidus: Yeah, it's more fun that way.

Emmanuel: Because I only want <u>good</u> people on my team.

Aniyah: Yeah, me too!

Kidus: Well that's not cool, I mean shouldn't everybody get to play?

Emmanuel: Yeah, it's just for fun, it's not like the basketball team or something.

Benson: Oh come on! I only want people who can really play on my team. Like, I don't want to end up with Emmanuel on my team; he shoots like a girl! Am I right?!

Benson laughs and looks around at everyone, but nobody laughs.

Emmanuel looks embarrassed and sad and the other kids look angry.

Aniyah: (Angrily) Dude!

Andrew: (Surprised) Dude!

Kidus: (Angrily) Dude!

Richard: (Calmly) Dude! Don't talk like that. That's offensive and mean.

Everybody except Benson nods in agreement

Andrew: Yeah. And I think that at recess, anybody who wants to play should get to play. When we're on teams, it's different.

Aniyah: I guess you're right. I mean it's fun to play with other kids who are good, but leaving kids out just because they aren't as good yet seems kind of mean.

Richard: I heard that there used to be a kid at this school who used a wheelchair.

Benson: Really?

Richard: Yeah, but the other kids didn't want him to be left out of everything so they found ways to include him in their games.

Aniyah: That's cool.

Emmanuel: I have asthma which makes it hard for me to breathe sometimes when I run around. I'm not really able to run fast enough to be on a team, but I still really like playing basketball. Recess is my only chance.

Benson: I never really thought of it like that.

Aniyah: Dude, I'll show you how girls shoot (pretends to shoot and swish!).

Richard: Whoa! Swish!

Kidus: That's right! (high fives Aniyah)

Benson: All right, you guys, I'm sorry. Come on, let's go play. We'll count off for teams.

Everybody: (Happily) Dude!! (high fives all around)

The End.

Lesson 31
Just Like Me

OBJECTIVES: Reinforce our common humanity

Build our sense of community

Engage students in mindfulness

Practice kindness

Assign final Peace Partners of the year

PREPARATION: Review lesson

Optional: bell or chime

Optional: student journals

This is our next to Peace of Mind class for the year. Our focus in this lesson is on community. We have been doing challenging work together for the last few weeks, but students have not been doing it alone. The activities in this lesson reinforce our common humanity and connection. We are all in this together.

Introduction

You might say: *Today is our next to last class. One of the best things for me about this year of Peace of Mind has been doing the work together in our class community. We all now have the same language for talking about managing our emotions, for solving conflicts, and for taking on some of the hardest work we can do - looking at our own biases and working for social justice. We can help each other remember that we have the tools to do this work, even when it's hard.*

Today we're going to do a partner activity that's about connection, and then do the Kindest things activity we did a few weeks ago. But first, let's start as we usually do.

Mindfulness Practice

Invite today's Mindful Leader(s) (ML) to come to the front of the class.

Prompt the ML to say: "Let's sit up a little straighter. Close your eyes or look down into your lap. Let's take 3 deep breaths."

Teacher Says: *Let your breath settle back into its natural rhythm. You don't have to change it at all.*

Say: *So remember, all I am going to say is See, Hear or Feel. You're going to try to move your attention around to focus on those things that you see, hear and feel. Don't worry if you get distracted and start thinking about something else. That's totally normal. As soon as you notice that your mind went somewhere else just try to start again. This might happen a bunch of times and that's fine.*

See… wait about ten seconds

Hear…. wait about ten seconds

Feel…. wait about ten seconds

Repeat this two or three times - if the students seem restless cut it shorter.

Okay, great job! Let's take one big deep breath and reach your arms up over your head as you breathe in and slowly float them down as you breathe out.

Optional: Ask ML to ring the bell.

Ask students to open their eyes and/or look up when they are ready.

Ask the ML to return to their seat(s).

1. **Just Like Me Partner Activity: A reminder of our common humanity**

   This is a powerful practice we first learned from author and educator <u>Tovi Hussein-Scruggs</u>, *President of the Coalition for Schools Educating Mindfully.*

   Have each person sit across from their Peace Partner (or another partner) either on the floor or in chairs. Sit knee to knee. Have your hands in your lap.

   Say: *I'm going to ask you to close your eyes or look down into your lap and listen to what I am saying. When I ask you to open your eyes, you can look into the eyes of the person sitting across from you or you can look at their hands in their lap.*

Invite the class to take 3 deep breaths.

Then say:

This person across from me wants to be happy. Just.. like.. me.. **Pause**

Open your eyes (they can choose to look each other in the eye or look at each other's hands)

Close your eyes or look down again

This person across from me has people that they care about. Just like me. **Pause**

Open your eyes (they can choose to look each other in the eye or look at each other's hands)

Close your eyes or look down again

This person across from me is worried about things. Just like me. **Pause**

Open your eyes (they can choose to look each other in the eye or look at each other's hands)

Close your eyes or look down again

This person across from me has dreams about their future. Just like me. **Pause**

Open your eyes (they can choose to look each other in the eye or look at each other's hands)

Close your eyes or look down again

This person across from me feels sad sometimes. Just like me. **Pause**

Open your eyes (they can choose to look each other in the eye or look at each other's hands)

Close your eyes or look down again

This person across from me feels like they don't fit in sometimes. Just like me. **Pause**

Open your eyes (they can choose to look each other in the eye or look at each other's hands)

Close your eyes or look down again

This person across from me is doing their best. Just like me. **Pause**

Open your eyes (they can choose to look each other in the eye or look at each other's hands)

Close your eyes or look down again

Okay, let's take a deep breath together.

End the practice.

Discuss

- What did that feel like for you?
- What did it feel like to look into the other person's eyes?
- What did it feel like to look at the other person's hands?
- What else can you think of that we all have in common?

2. Kindest Things Activity: Repeat from Lesson 20.

3. Kindness Chain Activity

Directions for the Class:

- Sit in a circle or as close to that as possible.
- Think of something kind to say about the person on your right.
- Take a moment to think about that person.

- We are not going to be talking about people's appearance so we won't be saying things like "I like your hair" or "your sweatshirt is cool."
- Instead, try to think about something that you know and admire about this person. Some examples could be "You make people laugh," "You always seem to try really hard," "I've noticed that you are a good friend to people," "You are very helpful," "You are great at drawing (or music, or math, or sports, etc.)."

> *NOTE: Some kids will feel uncomfortable with this activity so make sure to give students the opportunity to pass.*

You might say: *Sometimes, even if I'm sitting next to my best friend, my mind might go blank and I can't think of anything to say. If that happens to you just say that you need help and I'll choose someone else or I'll say something kind about that person myself. But we're all going to really try to do this.*

If they pass, you can ask for a volunteer to say something kind about this student.

After you go around the circle go back around the other way.

Alternate Kindness Chain Activity

If you think your students might not be comfortable saying these things in person, another way to do this is to have each student have a large index card taped to their back. Students can take turns going around and writing something kind on each person's card anonymously. Make sure to set expectations about kindness and give warnings about how joke comments can sometimes be misconstrued. Encourage earnest comments.

Discuss

- What did it feel like to say something kind about someone else?
- What did it feel like to have someone say something kind about you?
- If you did the face-to-face version of the activity: Did it feel uncomfortable in any way to give or receive these compliments? Why do you think that is?

Peace Partners

Give students time to share what they did for the Peace Partners.

Assign new Peace Partners. Remind your students that their job is to do at least one kind thing for their Peace Partner this week. This is the last Peace Partner you'll assign this year.

Closing words: *Okay, our time is up for today. Thank you for a great class, everyone.*

Optional: *Let's have a nice quiet moment for the bell. If you want to, you can close your eyes, picture your new Peace Partner, and imagine yourself doing something kind for them this week.*

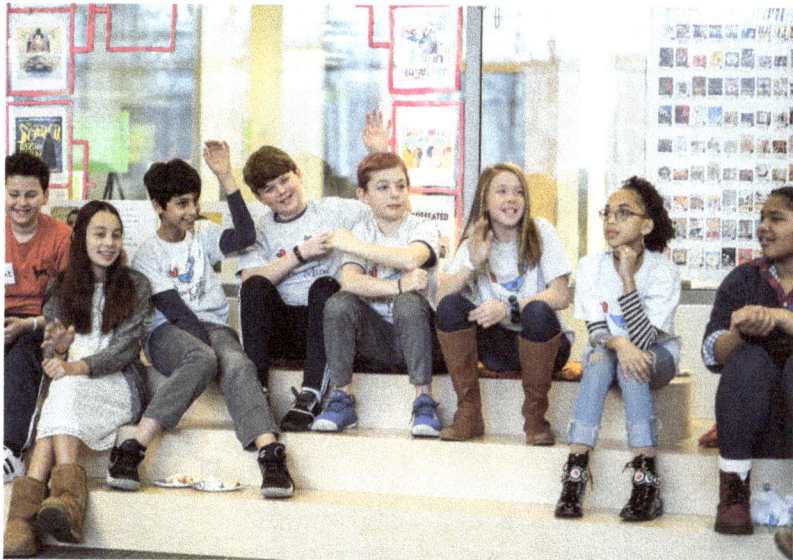

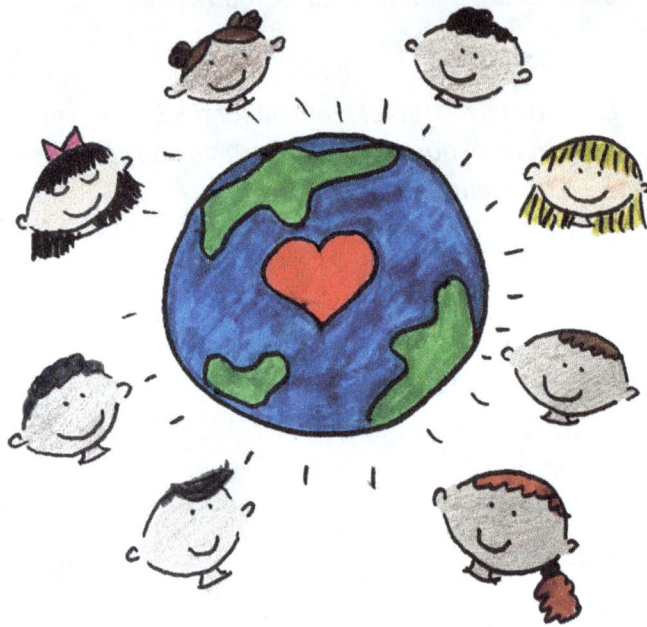

|

VI. Wrapping Up the Year

Lesson 32
Reflection and Next Steps Class

Objectives: Reflect and consider next steps

Engage students in mindfulness

Practice kindness

Preparation: Review lesson

Gather materials for reflection project

Optional: bell or chime

Optional: student journals

In his book *How to Be an Antiracist*, Ibram X. Kendi writes,

> *"The opposite of racist isn't 'not racist.' It is 'anti-racist.' … One either allows racial inequities to persevere, as a racist, or confronts racial inequities, as an anti-racist. There is no in-between safe space of 'not racist'"* (p. 9).

Kendi's call to action inspires us in our own work and inspires us to share this curriculum with you. If you have been teaching this curriculum all year, you have been helping your students build a powerful tool kit that they can use to become kinder and more compassionate people, to build healthy relationships, to engage in learning, to work for social change. What could be more important?

We invite you to close the year with this lesson reflecting with your students on what they have learned.

This reflection may lead to a class plan to co-design a service project in which they can put their skills to work. We leave it to you and your class to decide what will be the best expression of your students' learning and hopes. We've shared the project idea below to help you get the wheels turning.

Thank you for taking up this important work. The world so needs what you and your students have to give.

Mindfulness Practice

Invite your class to settle in for a mindful moment. Every student will now have many practices to draw on. Encourage everyone to choose their favorite practice, and practice together as a class for the final time this year.

Reflection

Take stock of the year with your students.

- Remind them that they know so much more about noticing and managing their emotions, about how their brains work, about the value of practicing kindness and empathy, about solving conflicts peacefully, and about their own identities than they may have known at the beginning of the year.
- Reflect on the conversations you have had exploring stereotypes, bias, and racism.
- Share your own reflections about how you have seen your students grow. What has impressed you? What has given you hope?

Ask: What is the most important thing you have learned in this class this year?

Ask: How could what you've learned in Peace class help to make your world more peaceful?

Ask: What do you want to do with the tools and insight you have gained this year to help yourself, your family, your community, your world?

Project

Invite your students into a writing, drawing or collage project that will allow students to answer these questions creatively.

These might be individual or small group projects, or even a class project with many interlocking pieces.

If this reflection produces the desire for greater action, consider a Capstone service project such as the one described below.

Peace Partners

Give students time to share what they did for their Peace Partners over the last week.

In Peace Partner Pairs, do the Gratitude Practice from Week 10, either focused on today or the whole year.

Closing words: *Thank you for a great year, everyone.*

Optional: *Let's have a nice quiet moment for the bell. If you want to, you can close your eyes and breathe, getting ready for whatever challenges and opportunities are ahead.*

NOTE FROM LINDA: Example of a Social Justice Capstone Project

One powerful way to help our students learn about history and privilege and identity is to make it personal.

At our school we recently learned from local historians that the very land that our school and adjacent park and recreation center had been built on had been stolen by the government from Black people in the 1930s. We invited the historians who uncovered this history as well as descendants of the original owners of the land to visit our school and talk to the kids about what happened.

After learning this history, my students began a letter-writing campaign to our Mayor and City Council to demand that the recreation center be renamed for the original owner, and that reparations be made to his family.

Taking Action

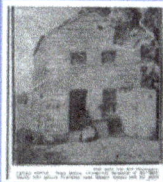

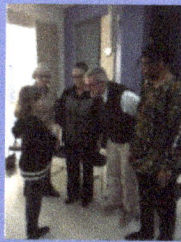

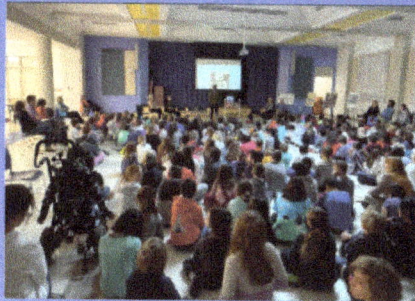

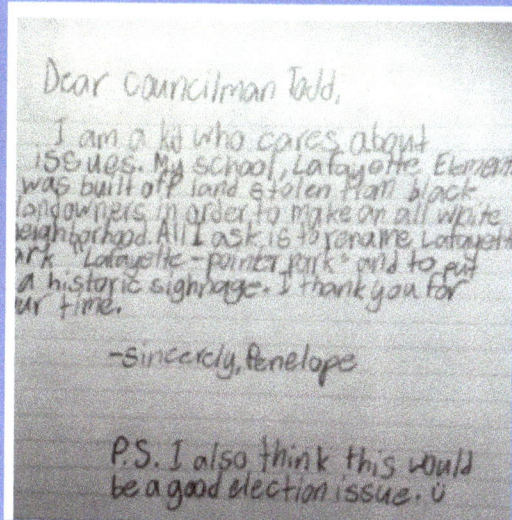

> Dear Councilman Todd,
>
> I am a kid who cares about issues. My school, Lafayette Elementary was built off land stolen from black landowners in order to make an all white neighborhood. All I ask is to rename Lafayette Park "Lafayette - painter park" and to put a historic sighnage. I thank you for ur time.
>
> —Sincerely, Penelope
>
> P.S. I also think this would be a good election issue. ☺

Sadly, it would be all too easy for educators in every part of the country to find stories similar to these - whether it be land stolen from people who were formerly enslaved or indigenous people. But these are issues our students care about and can engage in.

We hope hearing about this project inspires you to design one of your own!

– Peace Teacher Linda Ryden and Students at Lafayette ES, Washington DC

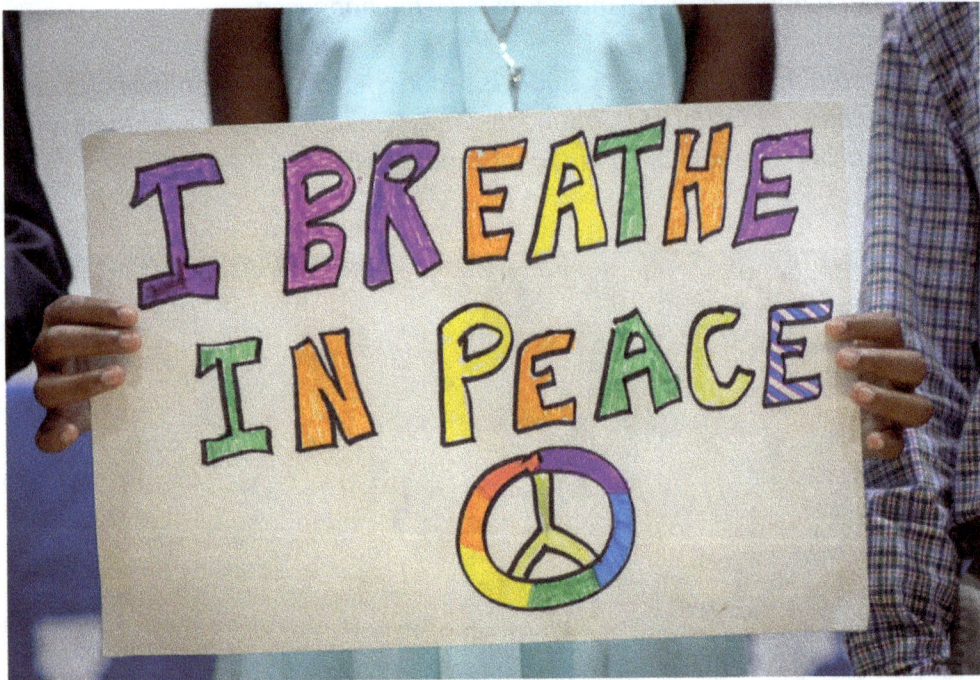

VII. Materials for Lessons

Materials for Lessons

Required

The only things you will definitely need for this curriculum are:

- a means to show videos to your class
- paper and writing materials for some lessons

Optional

Optional materials include:

- a journal for each student

- a bell or a chime

- collage materials

- Peace of Mind Tools and Resources

   — **The Conflict CAT Game**
   Peace of Mind created the Conflict CAT Game
   to help students integrate and apply skills they
   have been learning, including mindfulness
   practice, apologizing, and using tools to resolve
   conflicts. This game is optional - but very helpful
   and fun!

   — **Ways to Practice Mindfulness Poster**
   English / Spanish

   — **Brain Anchor Chart**

   — **Toolbox Anchor Chart**

   — **Mindfulness Practice Cards**
   English / Spanish

   All of these resources can be found
   at TeachPeaceofMind.org/shop/.

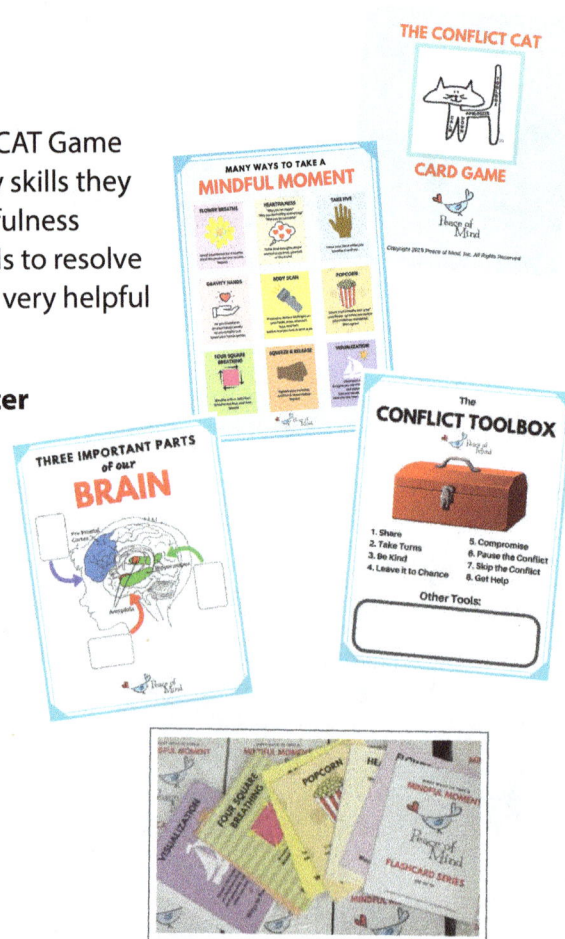

VIII. Resources

Social Justice Resources

Videos

"A Class That Turned Around Kids' Assumptions of Gender Roles!" Upworthy, September 1, 2016, https://www.youtube.com/watch?v=G3Aweo-74kY.

"Boys and Girls on Stereotypes". *NY Magazine*, March 7, 2018, https://www.youtube.com/watch?v=aTvGSstKd5Y.

Haymarket Books (2020, June 23) *Abolitionist Teaching and the Future of Our Schools* "A conversation with Bettina Love, Gholdy Muhammad, Dena Simmons and Brian Jones about abolitionist teaching and antiracist education." https://www.youtube.com/watch?v=uJZ3RPJ2rNc

Nick News (2020, June 29) *Kids, Race, and Unity | Hosted By Alicia Keys*

https://www.youtube.com/watch?v=OWsMEIODo6g "Hosted by Alicia Keys, Nick News talks with founders and leaders of the Black Lives Matter movement, offer tools for families to have constructive conversations about race, and highlights teen activists who are fighting racial injustice"

Spencer, John. http://bit.ly/spencervideos.

Uncomfortable Conversations with a Black Man (2020, June 3) In this video series, former NFL linebacker Emmanuel Acho's "sits down to have an "uncomfortable conversation" with white America, in order to educate and inform on racism, system racism, social injustice, rioting & the hurt African Americans are feeling today." https://www.youtube.com/watch?v=h8jUA7JBkF4&feature=youtu.be

Vox (2015 January 13) *The Myth of Race* "You may know exactly what race you are, but how would you prove it if somebody disagreed with you? Jenée Desmond Harris explains." https://www.youtube.com/watch?v=VnfKgffCZ7U.

Articles and Essays

ADL.org (2019, April) *How Should I Talk about Race in my Mostly White Classroom?* https://www.adl.org/education/resources/tools-and-strategies/how-should-i-talk-about-race-in-my-mostly-white-classroom

Hammond, Zaretta (2015, April 9) *Four Tools for Interrupting Implicit Bias.* https://crtandthebrain.com/four-tools-for-interrupting-implicit-bias/.

Landsman, Julie (2016, November) *Helping Students Discuss Race Openly.*
http://www.ascd.org/publications/educational-leadership/nov16/vol74/
num03/Helping-Students-Discuss-Race-Openly.aspx.

Madda, Mary Jo (2019) *Dena Simmons: Without Context Social Emotional
Learning Can Backfire.* EdSurge. https://www.edsurge.com/news/2019-05-15-
dena-simmons-without-context-social-emotional-learning-can-backfire

McIntosh, Peggy (1990) *White Privilege: Unpacking Invisible Knapsacks.*
Teaching Tolerance. https://www.tolerance.org/classroom-resources/texts/
white-privilege-unpacking-the-invisible-knapsack

Simmons, Dena (2019, April). *Why We Can't Afford Whitewashed Social-Emotional
Learning.* ASCD Education Update.
http://www.ascd.org/publications/newsletters/education_update/apr19/vol61/
num04/Why_We_Can't_Afford_Whitewashed_Social-Emotional_Learning.aspx

Simmons, Dena (2017, April 18) *How to Change the Story about Students of Color*
Dena Simmons explores how educators can inadvertently harm students of
color—and what we can do to bring out their best. *Greater Good Magazine*
https://greatergood.berkeley.edu/article/item/how_to_change_story_of_
students_of_color

Books

DiAngelo, Robin (2018) *White Fragility.* Beacon Press.
https://robindiangelo.com/publications/.

Hammond, Zaretta (2014) *Culturally Responsive Teaching and the Brain.* Corwin.
https://crtandthebrain.com/.

Kendi, Ibram X. (2017) Stamped from the Beginning : The Definitive History of
Racist Ideas in America. New York, NY, Nation Books.
https://www.ibramxkendi.com/.

Magee, Rhonda (2019) The Inner Work of Racial Justice. TarcherPerigee.
https://www.rhondavmagee.com/.

Oluo, Ijeoma So You Want to Talk About Race Seal Press, 2018.
http://www.ijeomaoluo.com/.

Teaching Tolerance. Let's Talk: Discussing Race, Racism and Other Difficult Topics with Students. http://www.tolerance.org/sites/default/files/general/TT%20Difficult%20Conversations%20web.pdf

Mindfulness and Brain Science Teaching Resources

Daniel Siegel's Brain Talk Video (YouTube)
http://www.drdansiegel.com/resources/everyday_mindsight_tools/

Breeding, K., & Harrison, J. (2007). *Connected and Respected: Lessons from the Resolving Conflict Creatively Program*. Cambridge, Mass.: Educators for Social Responsibility.

Hanson, Rick https://www.rickhanson.net/take-in-the-good/

Jennings, P. (2015). *Mindfulness for teachers: Simple skills for peace and productivity in the classroom*. The Norton Series on the Social Neuroscience of Education.

Jennings, P. A. (2019). *The Trauma-Sensitive Classroom: Building Resilience with Compassionate Teaching*. New York: W.W. Norton & Company.

Rechtschaffen, D., & Kabat-Zinn PhD, J. (2014). *The Way of Mindful Education: Cultivating Well-being in Teachers and Students*. Norton Books in Education.

Srinivasan, M. (2014). *Teach, Breathe, Learn: Mindfulness in and out of the Classroom*. Berkeley, CA: Parallax Press.

Treleaven, David (2018). *Trauma-Sensitive Mindfulness: Practices for Safe and Transformative Healing*. New York: W. W. Norton & Company.

Coaltion for Schools Educating Mindfully educatingmindfully.org.

Collaborative for Academic Social and Emotional Learning.
https://Casel.org

Greater Good Science Center at U.C. Berkeley. https://ggsc.berkeley.edu.

Center for Healthy Minds at the U. of Wisconsin https://centerhealthyminds.org/

Mindful Schools Resource Pages   http://www.mindfulschools.org/

Resources for Personal Mindfulness Practice and Well-being

Apps to Get You Started

Ten Percent Happier
Headspace
Calm

Good reads about developing a secular mindfulness practice

The Mindful Athlete by George Mumford

Hardwiring Happiness by Dr. Rick Hanson

Say What You Mean: A Mindful Approach to Nonviolent Communication by Oren Jay Sofer

Online Mindfulness Courses

Mindful Schools Courses for Educators   https://www.mindfulschools.org/

Elements of Meditation with Jeff Warren   https://jeffwarren.THiNKific.com/courses/

Unified Mindfulness   https://unifiedmindfulness.com

A few of the many wonderful Mindfulness Teachers out there to help you develop your practice (online or in person)

George Mumford
Mindfulness for Performance   https://georgemumford.com/

Sharon Salzberg
Real Love   https://www.sharonsalzberg.com

Sebene Selassie
Belonging and Identity   https://www.sebeneselassie.com

Jeff Warren   https://jeffwarren.org/

Home-School Connection

A September 2018 national study by Learning Heroes, *Developing Life Skills in Children: A Road Map for Communicating with Parents*, showed that 8 in 10 parents believe teaching and reinforcing social and emotional learning skills in school is very important.

Parents and guardians would like to count on schools as partners in teaching "life skills" to their children, and would like to be informed about what is being taught in Peace of Mind Class; we know from experience and from the Learning Heroes study that the two informants they trust most are their children and their children's teacher.

Here are a few things we hope you'll consider doing to build the bridge between home and school.

News from their children

Encourage your students to share what they have learned at home with trusted adults. Provide time in class to allow students to reflect on this sharing.

Newsletter

Send home a weekly or monthly newsletter with updates on what you are teaching in **Peace of Mind** Class. Parents and guardians appreciate knowing about the themes of the lessons you are teaching, and also the names of practices, such as Take Five Breathing, that they can ask their children to demonstrate for them at home.

Back to School Night

Offer information about **Peace of Mind** at Back to School Night. Please see the **Peace of Mind** website (TeachPeaceofMind.org) for materials that may be helpful to you in explaining the program. Photos and videos of your students practicing mindfulness can also be powerful tools to help parents understand what their children are learning.

Parent Evenings

Consider planning a mindfulness evening for parents during which they can experience some of the lessons and skills their children are learning. Introducing parents to the language of the curriculum can be helpful, too. Having a common language allows parents to prompt their children to use the skills they are learning at home.

You can find additional resources for parents on the **Peace of Mind** website at **TeachPeaceofMind.org.**

IX. Bibliography

Bradshaw, C. P. (2015). Translating research to practice in bullying prevention. American Psychologist, 70 (4), 322-332.

Breeding, K., & Harrison, J. (2007). *Connected and Respected: Lessons from the Resolving Conflict Creatively Program.* Cambridge, Mass.: Educators for Social Responsibility.

Chugh, Dr. Dolly (2018). *The Person You Mean to Be: How Good People Fight Bias.* New York, NY: Harper Business.

Csikszentmihalyi, Mihaly (2008) *Flow: The Psychology of Optimal Experience.* Harper Perennial Modern Classics.

Csikszentmihalyi, Mihaly (2004) *Flow: The Secret to Happiness.* TED, February 2004. https://www.ted.com/talks/mihaly_csikszentmihalyi_flow_the_secret_to_happiness?language=en

DiAngelo, Robin (2018) *White Fragility.* Beacon Press.

Durlak, J. A., Weissberg, R. P., Dymnicki, A. B., Taylor, R. D. & Schellinger, K. B. (2011). The impact of enhancing students' social and emotional learning: A meta-analysis of school-based universal interventions. Child Development, 82(1): 405–432.

Hammond, Zaretta (2014) *Culturally Responsive Teaching and the Brain.* Corwin.

Hammond, Zaretta. *Four Tools for Interrupting Implicit Bias.* Culturally Responsive Teaching and the Brain Website, April 9, 2015, https://crtandthebrain.com/four-tools-for-interrupting-implicit-bias/.

Hanson, R. (2015). *Hardwiring Happiness.* Random House USA.

Harris, Dan (2019) *10% Happier Revised Edition: How I Tamed the Voice in My Head, Reduced Stress Without Losing My Edge, and Found Self-Help That Actually Works--A True Story.* Dey Street Books.

Harris, Dan and Jeff Warren (2017) *Meditation for Fidgety Skeptics.* Spiegel & Grau

Harris, Jenée Desmond (2015). "The Myth of Race". Washington, DC: Vox. https://www.youtube.com/watch?v=VnfKgffCZ7U.

Haymarket Books (2020, June 23) *Abolitionist Teaching and the Future of Our Schools* Retrieved from: https://www.youtube.com/watch?v=uJZ3RPJ2rNc.

How Should I Talk about Race in my Mostly White Classroom? ADL.org, April 2019, https://www.adl.org/education/resources/tools-and-strategies/how-should-i-talk-about-race-in-my-mostly-white-classroom.

Jennings, P. (2015). *Mindfulness for teachers: Simple skills for peace and productivity in the classroom.* The Norton Series on the Social Neuroscience of Education.

Jennings, P. A. (2019). *The Trauma-Sensitive Classroom: Building Resilience with Compassionate Teaching.* New York: W.W. Norton & Company.

Kahneman, D. (2015). *Thinking, Fast and Slow.* New York: Farrar, Straus and Giroux.

Kendi, Ibram X. *Stamped from the Beginning: The Definitive History of Racist Ideas in America.* New York, NY, Nation Books, 2017.

Landsman, Julie. *Helping Students Discuss Race Openly.* ASCD.org, November 2016, http://www.ascd.org/publications/educational-leadership/nov16/vol74/num03/Helping-Students-Discuss-Race-Openly.aspx.

Lantieri, Linda. "How SEL and Mindfulness Can Work Together." Greater Good. April 7, 2015. Accessed September 28, 2015. Retrieved from: http://greatergood.berkeley.edu/article/item/how_social_emotional_learning_and_mindfulness_can_work_together.

Learning Heroes (2018, September) *Developing Life Skills in Children: A Road Map for Communicating with Parents.* Retrieved from: https://bealearninghero.org/parent-mindsets/

Lueke, A., & Gibson, B. (2015). Mindfulness Meditation Reduces Implicit Age and Race Bias: The Role of Reduced Automaticity of Responding. *Social Psychological and Personality Science*, 6(3), 284–291. https://doi.org/10.1177/1948550614559651

Madda, Mary Jo. *Dena Simmons: Without Context Social Emotional Learning Can Backfire.* EdSurge, May 15, 2019, https://www.edsurge.com/news/2019-05-15-dena-simmons-without-context-social-emotional-learning-can-backfire.

Magee, Rhonda (2019) *The Inner Work of Racial Justice.* TarcherPerigee.

Magee, Rhonda *How Mindfulness Can Defeat Racial Bias.* Greater Good Magazine, May 14, 2015.
https://greatergood.berkeley.edu/article/item/how_mindfulness_can_defeat_racial_bias

McIntosh, Peggy. *White Privilege: Unpacking Invisible Knapsacks.* Teaching Tolerance. 1989.
https://www.tolerance.org/classroom-resources/texts/white-privilege-unpacking-the-invisible-knapsack.

Menakem, Resmaa (2017) *My Grandmother's Hands.* Central Recovery Press.

Metz, S.M., Frank, J.L., Reibel, D., Cantrell, T., Sanders, R., & Broderick, P.C. (2013). The effectiveness of Learning to BREATHE program on adolescent emotion regulation. *Research in Human Development, 10*(3), 252-272.

Mumford, George (2015) *The Mindful Athlete: Secrets to Pure Performance.* Parallax Press.

Nick News, *Kids, Race, and Unity | Hosted By Alicia Keys.* June 29, 2020,
https://www.youtube.com/watch?v=OWsMElODo6g.

O'Brennan, L., & Bradshaw, C. (2013). *School Climate: A Research Brief.* A report prepared for the National Education Association, Washington, DC.

Oluo, Ijeoma *So You Want to Talk About Race* Seal Press, 2018.

Rechtschaffen, D., & Kabat-Zinn PhD, J. (2014). *The Way of Mindful Education: Cultivating Well-being in Teachers and Students.* Norton Books in Education.

Schonert-Reichl, K. A., & Lawlor, M. S. (2010). The effects of a mindfulness-based education program on pre-and early adolescents' well-being and social and emotional competence. *Mindfulness, 1*(3), 137-151.

Schonert-Reichl, K. A., Oberle, E., Lawlor, M. S., Abbott, D., Thomson, K., Oberlander, T. F., & Diamond, A. (2015). Enhancing cognitive and social–emotional development through a simple-to-administer mindfulness-based school program for elementary school children: A randomized controlled trial. *Developmental Psychology, 51*(1), 52-66.

Seppala, E., Simon-Thomas, E., Brown, S. L., Worline, M. C., Cameron, C. D., & Doty, J. R. (2017). *The Oxford Handbook of Compassion Science*. New York, NY: Oxford University Press.

Siegel, D. J., & Bryson, T. P. (2012). *The Whole-Brain Child*. London: Constable & Robinson.

Simmons, Dena. *Why We Can't Afford Whitewashed Social-Emotional Learning*. ACSD.org, April 2019, http://www.ascd.org/publications/newsletters/education_update/apr19/vol61/num04.

Simmons, Dena (2017, April 18) *How to Change the Story about Students of Color*

Retrieved from *Greater Good Magazine* https://greatergood.berkeley.edu/article/item/how_to_change_story_of_students_of_color

Sofer, Oren Jay (2018). Say What You Mean: A Mindful Approach to Nonviolent Communication. Shambhala Press.

Srinivasan, M. (2014). *Teach, Breathe, Learn: Mindfulness in and out of the Classroom*. Berkeley, CA: Parallax Press.

Tatum, Dr. Beverly Daniel (2017). *Why Are All the Black Kids Sitting Together in the Cafeteria?: And Other Conversations About Race*. New York, NY: Basic Books.

Teaching Tolerance. *Let's Talk: Discussing Race, Racism and Other Difficult Topics with Students*. Accessed July 30, 2020, http://www.tolerance.org/sites/default/files/general/TT%20Difficult%20Conversations%20web.pdf.

Treleaven, David (2018). *Trauma-Sensitive Mindfulness: Practices for Safe and Transformative Healing*. New York: W. W. Norton & Company.

Weare, K. (2013). Developing mindfulness with children and young people: A review of the evidence and policy context. *Journal of Children's Services, 8(2)*, 141-153.

Zoogman, S., Goldberg, S.B., Hoyt, W.T., & Miller, L. (2015). Mindfulness interventions with youth: A meta-analysis. *Mindfulness, 6*, 290 - 302.

Zenner, C., Hermleben-Kurz, S., & Walach, H. (2014). Mindfulness-based interventions in schools: A systematic review and meta-analysis. *Frontiers in Psychology, 5*, article 603.

X. Credits

Hand Model of the Brain: Dr. Dan Siegel's *Hand Model of the Brain*. (2018) Found at https://www.youtube.com/watch?v=f-m2YcdMdFw. Mind Your Brain, Inc. Used with permission. All rights reserved.

Identity Maps: Mapping Your Identity: A Back-to-School Ice Breaker : Lesson Plans

"See, Hear, Feel": Shinzen Young, Unified Mindfulness. Unifiedmindfulness.com

The Conflict Escalator: Kreidler, William J., *Teaching Conflict Resolution through Children's Literature*. New York: Scholastic Professional Books, 1994

The THiNK Test: TOP 16 QUOTES BY BERNARD MELTZER: A-Z Quotes. (n.d.). Retrieved from https://www.azquotes.com/author/9957-Bernard_Meltzer

Children's Photos: Stacy Beck Photography and LNJ Designs Photo

Drawings: Linda Ryden

XI. Appreciation

This curriculum, like everything we do, is inspired by my students and my teachers. Each one of the more than 1,000 children I have worked with at Lafayette Elementary School in Washington, DC, has taught me something important, and some have left lasting imprints on my heart. I am especially grateful to my students who joined SPARK Club (Students Planning a Revolution of Kindness) who helped me to create the equity-inspired lessons in this curriculum. Their honesty, openness, and dedication to creating a more peaceful, just world makes me feel hopeful in a time when hope is hard to find.

This curriculum would never have happened without Megan Vroman, Principal of Ida B. Wells Middle School in Washington, DC who asked us to create a Peace of Mind curriculum for her students that would be a cornerstone of the new school she was opening. We were so honored to be part of Principal Vroman's vision and we are so grateful to her, her staff and her students for their willingness to pilot this curriculum. Their support, feedback and cooperation have made this a much stronger offering.

Dr William Blake, Director of SEL for DC Public Schools, has been steady in his support, keynoting our conference and believing in our program. Krystal Butler and Bode Aking, DCPS SEL Specialists, have shown their dedication by showing up at Peace of Mind events big and small, making such important contributions despite their truly challenging jobs. We are really so grateful!

This curriculum is inspired by so many wonderful meditation teachers - some who know they are my teachers and some who do not. I have learned so much from Jeff Warren, Dan Harris, Sebene Selassie, Oren Jay Sofer, Rick Hanson, Sharon Salzberg, Jay Michelson and many others. Many thanks to all of you for so freely sharing your wisdom.

As a white woman, writing lessons about racial justice was challenging at times. I am indebted to the teachers who helped me to find my way through. These teachers include Dena Simmons, Bettina Love, Gholdy Muhammed, Liz Kleinrock, Tovi Scruggs-Hussein, Grace Helms Kotre, Sally Albright Green, Ijeoma Oluo, Dr. Ibram X. Kendi, Verna Myers, Zaretta Hammond, Resmaa Menakem, Lama Rod Owens, Rhonda Magee, and many others. I am so grateful to be working during such a moment rich in Critical Race Theory and revolutionary thinkers.

I'd like to thank the people who have been there to support Peace of Mind in everything we do, big or small from the beginning. Our dedicated Board of Directors, Elizabeth Whisnant, Subrat Biswal, Chapin Springer, Darrel Jodrey, and Elizabeth Hoffman, have been creative, supportive and fierce advocates for our work. Harriet Sanford, Jackie Wright Snowden, David Trachtenberg, Avideh Shashaani, Jelena Popovich, Shawn Donnelly, Russell and Stefanie Wallach, and Rie Odsbjerg Werner have been wonderful ambassadors for Peace of Mind, providing support and opening doors in so many important ways.

Peace of Mind Inc is a small nonprofit organization. We literally could not do this work without the generous support of our funders: The NEA Foundation, the Bender Foundation, the Fund for the Future of our Children, and over 100 individual donors who keep the Peace of Mind mission alive.

We are grateful for the help we have received in putting together this curriculum in big and small ways. Madeleine Sagebiel has been an outstanding intern, always willing to do the detail work and also to offer big ideas when needed. My son, Henry Cohen contributed the lesson on Flow and has continued to expand my knowledge of meditation and mindfulness through his travels to the "deep end." My daughter Rosemary, a social justice warrior, always keeps me on my toes and pushes me to see new perspectives. Krystal Butler and Bode Aking, SEL Specialists with the DC Public Schools, showed true dedication by showing up at everything we did -- events or meetings big and small -- always making such important contributions in the midst of their truly challenging jobs. My sister, Dr. Patricia Ryden generously shared her background in media literacy to help to create the lessons in Unit 6. She is the Ben Hogan of sisters.

As always, I am grateful to the Principal of Lafayette Elementary School, Dr. Carrie Broquard, for believing in Peace of Mind enough to give me a spot on the very full Master Schedule and a beautiful Peace Room to work from. The opportunity to have freedom to grow, experiment and create is increasingly rare in public schools today and I am very grateful for that gift.

There is one person who makes Peace of Mind possible more than any other and that is my friend, partner and Peace of Mind Executive Director, Cheryl Cole Dodwell. Cheryl is a one-woman, non-profit miracle. Since I am teaching full-time and not good for much more than the content of the lessons, she somehow manages to be everything else at once. While running our small non-profit single-handedly, she is also the most thoughtful, detail-oriented editor and publisher. She is truly a co-author on this and all of our curricula. None of this would happen without her tireless, unrelenting commitment. Cheryl's dedication to helping children, making the world a better, kinder place, and her innate goodness, decency and integrity are the magic behind Peace of Mind. There are never going to be enough words to express my gratitude.

Linda
July 2020

About Linda Ryden, Teacher and Author

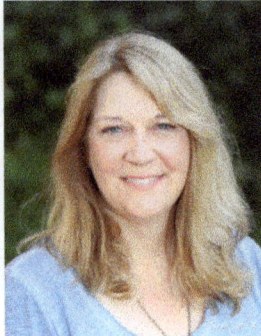

Linda Ryden is the creator of the Peace of Mind Program, a cutting edge combination of mindfulness, conflict resolution, social emotional learning and equity. Linda is the author of the Peace of Mind Curriculum Series and is the full-time Peace Teacher at Lafayette Elementary School, a public school in Washington, DC, where she teaches weekly Peace of Mind classes to more than 700 children.

Linda is the author of several children's books, including *Henry is Kind, Sergio Sees the Good*, and *Tyaja Uses the THiNK Test* all published by Tilbury House Publishers and *Rosie's Brain* published by Peace of Mind Press. *Rosie's Brain* has recently been translated into Spanish and is available as "El Cerebro de Rosita."

Linda has had several articles published in *The Washington Post* including "My Students Call Me the Peace Teacher." Her work has been featured in *The Huffington Post, The Washington Post, Washingtonian Magazine, Washington Parent, Washington Family,* EdSurge, and Edutopia. Linda recently gave a keynote speech to the National Network of State Teachers of the Year about mindfulness and racial justice.

Linda is the founder of Peace of Mind Inc, a 501c3 nonprofit organization that supports educators in teaching mindfulness, neuroscience, social emotional learning, conflict resolution and social justice to support our students and move our schools toward equity and racial justice.

Linda brings a passion for teaching peace and over 25 years of teaching experience to her work with children and adults. Linda lives in Washington D.C. with her husband Jeremiah Cohen, owner of Bullfrog Bagels, their two children, and their dog Phoebe. TeachPeaceofMind.org

About Cheryl Cole Dodwell

Cheryl Cole Dodwell is the co-author of the *Peace of Mind Core Curricula* for Grades 1 and 2, Grades 3-5, Grades 4 and 5, and Middle School. She oversees the development of the *Peace of Mind Curriculum Series*, *Henry and Friends Storybook Series* and other Peace of Mind resources. Cheryl brings dedication and passion, a love of writing and editing, a background in finance and publishing, and deep experience in mindfulness, healing work and parenting to her work as Executive Director of Peace of Mind Inc. She is grateful to be able to contribute through Peace of Mind to making our world a kinder, more supportive, anti-racist and inclusive place for all. TeachPeaceofMind.org.

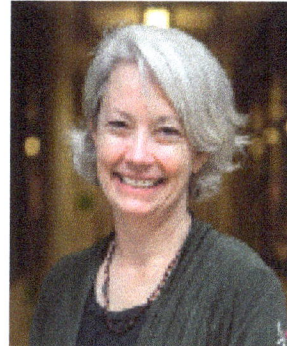